I0570170

50 And Fabulous

Navigating Wrinkles, Spasms and Generational Chasms

50 And Fabulous

Navigating Wrinkles, Spasms and Generational Chasms

Publisher: Rampant Feline Media/Betsy Chasse www.betsychasse.net

© 2024 All Rights Reserved

ISBN Paperback: 979-8-9910714-0-6

ISBN Kindle: 979-8-9910714-1-3

Table of Contents

Introduction

By Betsy Chasse

I arrived in my 50s, hopeful and excited for the next phase of my life's journey.

The world had other plans. My birthday happened about a week before the world shut down and went into hiding and all the plans I had made evaporated into thin air.

I was given a year to contemplate my life in a way I'm not sure I was prepared for or really wanted to do.

To say that I am not where I expected to be is an understatement. And to acknowledge that my 50s feel a little bit like the cosmic joke and less like the free-wheeling wild adventure I was expecting.

I suppose, regardless of your gender, realizing your body is aging yet your mind still twists and turns like the younger version of yourself. Still yearning for love, dreaming of future plans, but now hoping I make it long enough to experience them.

I realized I had questions, a lot of them and in a conversation with my dear friend Claudia I realized the best way to get the answers I seek was to ask and share those answers with you.

And so here we are with a wonderful collaboration of amazing women and one man ironically. My intention was not to fill this book with only women, but I wanted to fill this book with people who had wisdom that was valuable and worth sharing and so yes, the most wonderful group of women showed up and so did my dear friend Gregory.

I learned a lot from these writers, some of which I already thought I knew, but needed a reminder and a perspective that shifts as we age and some new tidbits that offered me peace and a release from the fears that I had about what this next phase of my journey will look like.

I know you will find that too in the pages of this book.

Welcome to the next, but not the end, a new beginning.

Forward

by Claudia Micco

"The afternoon knows what the morning never suspected"

- Robert Frost

The march of time is a relentless force, one that we can never truly escape. As women, we are thrust into this journey from the moment we are born, constantly navigating uncertain paths and facing impossible decisions about our bodies, relationships, careers, and motherhood. Society demands that we have it all figured out by a certain age, but just when we start to feel confident and in control, time throws us curveballs and shakes our foundations. Our bodies morph and change in ways that no one ever warned us about or adequately prepared us for. We make jokes about growing older, but it's not until we reach old age that we fully grasp the weight of it all. The very concept of gravity takes on a whole new meaning after 50. And it's not just physical changes that blindside us; societal expectations and restrictions are placed upon aging women, making us question the ground we thought was stable beneath our feet. Relationships shift, friends and loved ones pass away, and the world continues to evolve at a dizzying pace. It's a confusing dilemma - once thinking old people were strange and smelly, now realizing that we ourselves are becoming "weird" and "smelly." But they don't tell us that while our hearts may still feel young and vibrant, the mirror tells a different story. The stark contrast between mind and body can be simultaneously overwhelming and comical. The journey of time is one filled with unexpected twists and turns that can leave us feeling both exhilarated and exhausted as we try to keep up with its unrelenting pace.

The burning desire to create a compilation of unique stories has consumed me for years. These tales are not for the faint of heart - they will make you laugh, scream in terror, and feel uplifted, but above all else, they are deeply personal. Within these pages, you will find a mix of life experiences and practical advice from experts like doctors, writers, lawyers, personal coaches, professors, and authors who have become dear friends. But it was Betsy Chasse, the brilliant creator and visionary, who approved this project without hesitation. Her platform allows us to share our heartfelt stories and showcase the brilliance of each author. As you dive into these pages, you will experience each writer's raw emotions and unique perspectives as they navigate through life's unpredictable changes. This is not just a book about hot flashes - it delves into all the unexpected transformations that come with this stage in life, ones that every reader will undoubtedly relate to on a personal level.

With each turn of the page, the authors in this book reveal raw and gritty truths about the journey into middle age. They offer hard-hitting advice on the critical importance of specific types of exercise - from grueling strength training to whole-body vibration that shakes one's core. Other writers delve deeply into the social implications of this pivotal phase, predicting the seismic shifts we can anticipate as we march forward. Still, others share their harrowing personal tales, revealing how they rose above societal expectations and shattered barriers to forge their own unique paths. As I read these powerful anecdotes, I am filled with immense gratitude and honor to be a part of such a transformative collection. In this book, you will undoubtedly see fragments of your own story reflected in the stories of these brave and resilient authors.

We all strive to find a balance between being likable and maintaining our sanity. A true leader, someone in control of their destiny, understands the importance of solitude and self-reflection in honing skills and perfecting strategies. During these moments of isolation, one can emerge more robust and more determined than ever. I applaud the authors for opening up about these pivotal moments in their lives at 50.

Get ready to dive into the unvarnished truth about life in the second half—no sugar-coating, no coddling. These are real stories from real people who have been through it all and lived to tell the tale. So buckle up and take notes because this is wisdom you won't find in any self-help book or Instagram quote. We're getting down and dirty with the good, bad, and ugly of what it means to live life after 50.

Chapter One
The Grandmother Tree
by Kerri Hummingbird Sami

There once was a Medicine Woman who felt the call of The Grandmother Tree who whispered in her ear, "Your time is coming, dear one. Prepare."

Except, the Medicine Woman was not a Medicine Woman yet. She was a maiden in distress, seeking love and validation from anyone who could comfort her that she was still young and desirable. When she gazed at herself in the mirror, she felt distressed by the wrinkles appearing on her face and by the sagging of her breasts from breastfeeding her boys. No matter how many marathons she ran, she could not outrun Time.

The Grandmother Tree called to her heart: "This is not who you are. Take a look around you."

When she looked around her, she saw that her two young sons needed direction. She saw the ugly truth seeping through her rose-colored glasses, and she saw with clarity the example of mother, woman, and adult that she was setting for her boys. She was no longer a pretty maiden; she was a young mother resisting the depth and breadth of motherhood. She was burying herself in bottles of wine and distractions–anything to feel good, yet feeling worse every day. She was paying therapists every week to listen to her complain about her life and refusing to make the changes she needed to make.

She was blaming her partner, her parents, and her friends; the fingers pointed everywhere but to herself. All of this self-awareness was an overwhelming dose of truth. It finally clicked inside: I can't keep going this way.

The Grandmother Tree encouraged her: "You are so much more than this. Let yourself become who you are in truth."

And so the Medicine Woman, who was not yet a Medicine Woman, left the gilded cage of illusions with its masks and seductions and comfortable miseries and followed the call of The Grandmother Tree in a leap of faith. She left behind her husband, her home, her financial security, and her story of woe. She set out on a new adventure of discovery with her sons and hoped that things would get better. I mean, how could it get any worse? She asked herself.

She found herself in the desert surrounded by cacti, each one with a thorn that pricked her awake in new and unexpected ways. Each thorn punctured her false reality and called her forth with self-awareness to make new choices and become resilient and wise. No longer could she blame anyone else for the conditions of her life: the cactus pricked her every time she succumbed to feeling weak, helpless, and ungrateful.

The Grandmother Tree whispered: "Show your boys how to be truthful, authentic, grateful, and self-empowered. You first."

For years, the Medicine Woman, who was now becoming a Medicine Woman, wandered in that desert filled with cactus, and there were times that she wanted to lie down and die. She wanted to give up and be rescued by a knight in shining armor. Except there were no knights to be found. There were just more cactus pricks urging her to wake up from the delusion that anyone else could rescue her from her life and choices. She was being called forth by The Grandmother Tree to dig into her initiations and become strong and resilient through them for herself and her sons.

Perhaps because of stubbornness and the need to prove she was right, she stood up time and time again in that field of cacti and kept going. She became extremely resourceful. She learned her lessons well from that desert, and she began to cultivate something deep within herself: compassion.

As the mental chatter and self-judgments diminished with her presence and self-compassion, she began to hear the wisdom of The Grandmother Tree more clearly.

"Let their father lavish them with money, gifts, and travel. You can lavish them with love, compassion, and acceptance," the Grandmother Tree whispered to her heart. "Trust yourself."

The Medicine Woman was now firmly on her golden path of unconditional love, and every cactus prick became a new gleaming gold nugget of wisdom to place in her heart. As she learned to trust the wisdom of her heart, she guided her boys through the thorny patches of entitlement, disrespect for the feminine, manipulation, dishonesty, greed, and anger and resentment that she wasn't playing the role assigned to her.

She taught her boys The Four Agreements and practiced them daily in every interaction: Be Impeccable with Your Word, Don't Take Anything Personally, Don't Make Assumptions, and Do Your Best. To teach these powerful agreements to her sons, she had to live them herself. There was no longer "Do what I say, not what I do" of her parent's generation. Nope. Those days were gone. If she was going to teach her sons to live by the agreements, the best way was through demonstration.

When the Medicine Woman detected false conditioning or negative energy seeping into her home, she whipped out her sage and cleared the space. When she felt disrespected, she healed herself of the wounded place within. She used everything that hooked her attention into self-judgment and self-doubt to reclaim more of her inner power and trust herself. Little by little, the Medicine Woman claimed total responsibility for her life, her dream, and the impact of her mothering on her sons. She no longer expected anyone to love her and honor her path: she loved herself unconditionally and honored her own path to sovereignty.

11

The journey through the desert of prickly cacti transformed the Medicine Woman, and her heart and home became a space of unconditional love and acceptance. Through careful consideration and mindfulness, the Medicine Woman cultivated an oasis in her home—a safe space of compassion where breakdown led to breakthrough. Each member of the family was called forth to do their own soul work, and the Medicine Woman practiced not fixing other people's lives. She did her inner work to accept everyone just the way they were while offering silent prayers of gratitude and certainty in the worth of all of her family members. There were days she was sorely tested in this lesson, and her heart cracked open with grief to witness the paths her children chose to walk.

The Medicine Woman proactively filled her home with love and prayer, inviting the Divine into every aspect of her life and home. She minded how she used her Word to leave it open for current circumstances to shift and beneficial outcomes to result...no matter how messy it looked in the moment. She did her inner work to accept her children through their soul lessons and keep opening her heart in more compassion. Sometimes, her children felt dark, depressed, and dense with the fog of self-loathing. It was hard for the Medicine Woman to feel this; she wished it would change, and sometimes she felt like a failure as a mother.

The Grandmother Tree whispered to her: "Where there is great love, there is safety to be as you are...shadows and all. Expressing these shadows is a sign that you have made a space of great love."

The Medicine Woman listened to this guidance and began to realize that it was a blessing that her children felt safe to take off the masks of perfection and be real with how they really felt. She put into the bonfire the old dream of family pictures where everyone was smiling and happy and doing what was expected of them (while secretly hating every moment of pretending). She desired instead a family portrait where everyone was authentic and fulfilled and walking to the beat of their own drums.

As her home life filled with love and grace, pricks from cactus were easier to move through. Her children began leaving home to venture off into the great wilderness and have their own adventures, and the Medicine Woman wondered what was next for her in the wake of their departures.

She began to realize that the lessons learned from her journey were helpful to others, and so the Medicine Woman started sharing them. She knew enough from her own journey of being a mother that only those who really yearned for her wisdom would listen to what she had to offer. There were a few more prickly cactus on the road to become a messenger and mentor, and she took each prick with grace and gratitude for how that encounter gave her the wisdom to become masterful.

A few years into this journey, after she had good success with being a messenger and mentor, the Medicine Woman took a walk through the woods to relax. She decided to sit down next to the river and meditate. As everything became still and quiet, she closed her eyes and turned within to listen to her Spirit. A vision of a hollow bone appeared in her mind's eye. She saw how the bone had no more marrow, nothing blocking the inside, and so energy could freely pass through it.

"You will become a hollow bone," whispered The Grandmother Tree, "and the marrow you must release is your story, your identity, your opinions and perspectives. Practice humility."

The Medicine Woman had grown fond of herself with self-love and self-compassion, and she didn't really like this idea. She had made a good life for herself and was able to offer her wisdom to others by sharing her story and her perspective. She was helping people. Why would she give all of that up?

The Grandmother Tree whispered, "You have a greater calling to help others find their own answers without giving them yours."

The Medicine Woman felt this truth sink deep into her heart. She knew that everyone had a unique thumbprint that no one before, and no one after, would ever have. She knew that it was on purpose that each thumbprint was unique for a one-time-ever life journey. And she also knew that the best answers were the ones found within.

13

What people really need, the Medicine Woman considered, is a shady place to lean against and contemplate life where it's safe to sit for a while without being bothered, and where it's safe to sleep and dream until rested.

And just as she had that realization, a bridge stretched before her over a deep bottomless chasm. On the other side of the bridge she could see a giant blossoming tree with a thick trunk and branches gracefully reaching out in every direction. She could smell the heavenly fragrance of the flowers wafting on the winds. The sun was glowing behind the great tree, the breeze was gentle and mild, and the meadow around the tree looked soft to sit on while leaning against the tree.

"This is who you are meant to be," whispered The Grandmother Tree. "To claim that for yourself, to be the gift you are, simply cross the bridge and let go of yourself."

The Medicine Woman felt so much fear it made her tremble. Will I die? she wondered. What will happen to me?

The Grandmother Tree heard her fears echoing on the winds and whispered, "You will die anyway. This is your chance to blossom into your greatest potential."

To comfort herself, the Medicine Woman placed a hand on her heart, a hand on her belly, and took three deep belly breaths. She felt a Sacred Yes in her heart and knew what she had to do.

The Medicine Woman mustered her courage and took the first step onto the bridge.

For my chapter, I share a practice of writing The Mythic Story, which has four parts:

- The WakeUp Call
- The Great Departure
- The Vision Quest
- The Bid for Power

14

I invite Inner Medicine students to open sacred space, set intention for the Mythic Story, and then pull four oracle cards. For my Mythic Story, I used The Shaman's Dream oracle deck by Alberto Villoldo and Colette Baron-Reid. The cards I pulled were: 29 - Horned Cactus, Resourcefulness, 27 - Heart Home, Compassion, 28 - Hollow Bone, Teachability, and 54 - The Crossing, Initiation.

Spirit did a wonderful job at pointing me in the right direction to share some wisdom for this book. Many blessings on your journey of self-discovery.

About Kerri Hummingbird Sami

Kerri Hummingbird Sami, Medicine Woman, Mother, and Mentor, is the Founder of Inner Medicine Training, a Mystery School that shares potent ancient traditions from the Andes and Himalayas for owning your wisdom and living your purpose. She is the #1 internationally best-selling author of "Inner Medicine: Becoming One with Mother Earth for the Survival of Humanity," "Love Is Fierce: Healing the Mother Wound," "The Second Wave: Transcending the Human Drama" (on the International Bestseller charts for over 250 weeks!) and the award-winning best-selling book "Awakening To Me: One Woman's Journey To Self Love" which describes the early years of her spiritual awakening. As the host of Soul Nectar Show, Ms. Hummingbird inspires people to lead their lives wide awake with an authenticity, passion, and purpose that positively impacts others. As a healer and mentor, she catalyzes mind shifts that transform life challenges into gifts of wisdom.

Chapter Two
50 Years to Dream: A New Dream
by Rebecka Gregory

Rolling into 50 is a moment one has to reflect on where they have been. It is a surreal feeling of the journey you have been on and where you are at this point. Living in a dream that begins to fade as you begin to explore where you desire to go and who you wish to be. It's like being a kid again and moving back into the wonderment of life with a new set of tools; at least, this was my experience. An opening of changes in your body, mind, and soul of this life you have lived thus far and how you wish to continue. A creation of a new dream, a new you, and a new way to be if you choose. Turning 50 for me, I remember I told everyone that I was one and got to start over. I get to create how I wish to be now with a new sense of wisdom learned from this road I have traveled thus far. Looking back, yet not anchoring into the past, I am opening to healing, learning, forgiving, and letting go of all that does not fit this new version of me that I dream of creating. Now, there is also adjusting to changes in the body that can be challenging to move through, such as wearing reading glasses; I thought that was a myth; no, it is real. New aches popping up from the wear and tear I put on my body. This new change is all part of the process of becoming grounded in who you are: body, mind, and soul. This new beginning is really all about opening to receive a new cycle of you if you choose and are ready to heal the past to claim you.

Trucking along the path to 50 and all that I experienced in my life, I had to reflect on the trials and tribulations that I have put myself through. I had to look at the places that I hid from leftovers from childhood hurt and pain. I had to see the truth of the path I chose to live and take responsibility for all of it. Yes, others might have played a huge role in the experience. The bottom line is that was it only a reflection of the inner truth that I was hiding from, facing, reflecting on, or just completely in denial? I have learned along the way this reflection is real and part of us all—the outer guidance for us to find who we wish to be by looking in. The universe is always showing us everything we require to succeed in this world. It is just taking the time and moments to see them. We live in a constant dream state, redirecting our world to open, expand, and grow. Or stay stuck in the dream of despair, suffering, and hopelessness. It is a world we chose, and when you turn 50, the game is on. It is now a new milestone to 100, and how will you get there?

Now moving towards 55, I have had five years in this state of 50, and things have been fabulous and challenging at the same time. Looking at all these pieces of myself and unraveling them is not for the faint of heart at all. It will test you to the core of you. There will be days when you are on top of the world and days when everything comes to a head; you are curled in a ball, crying tears you did not know you had. I invite you to embrace yourself, whatever it looks like. For turning 50, you start to move into this learning to un-trick yourself from the fuckery you have been telling yourself and dealing with others, yet also working thru reprograming all the lies you have lived with thus far. Loving others and loving yourself is huge. That is the key I found in this life transition; it is all about learning to love myself. My whole life, I have allowed the world to drain me, caring for others, worrying for others, and wanting to fix everyone so they are happy. Guess who wasn't? Yes me. I gave all of myself to the world and left nothing for me. So now I am learning to take care of me. I still have a long way to go; however, each day I wake up, I get closer to feeling like I am living a life of self-love, self-care, and inner wonderment of my fabulousness of me. Looking back, you must laugh at all we have to go through to get here to this place, and if you knew this earlier, how different your life would be. Then, we realize this is a life that we come here to live to feel deeply all the emotions that the world must experience. My world is now moving into experiencing love, joy, and happiness by learning to detach from all that does not bring that. That is how I desire to end my dream in this life—living a full life of experiencing it all. For doesn't it all work together? It is a beautiful dance of life. If we do not experience the dark parts, then we will never appreciate the light of life that spirals as part of our existence to our next dance after death.

Living now, the question I ask myself is, does this honor me and bring joy in my heart? If it does not, that leads me to explore why or just say no. I have learned that sometimes, I just need to sit back and allow all the pieces to unfold before moving forward for that to be right. A perfect example is my move; I just made it to the mountains. My call from the beach to the mountains has been a journey that started right before I turned 50. I went on a five-year exploration, traveling the mountain towns, looking for a place to call home. I knew it had to be a place that made my heart sing, and it was going to take some time, yet part of me was not open to accept that at all. I wanted it now. I felt like a little girl who turned into a blueberry in Willy Wonka and did not want to wait. Somehow, I tamed that little brat part of me and waited and waited until the time was right for all to unfold, and boy, did it. I remember the day I was reminded what the feeling of joy and where you belong really was. I had forgotten that true feeling in my heart, the one of home. That was until I drove through a little mountain town in Alabama, and my heart blew open, tears ran down my face, and this swell of love and joy came rushing over me, and I knew I was home. This was the place for me. The joy inside me could not be contained, yet I knew I also had to wait for the right place to open. I had to listen to my heart and wait until the right time for all the pieces to line up. When all was aligned and ready, we found our home, sold our home, and moved within 90 days. And once again, when I drove on this property, I began to cry and knew this is home, and I am home here… So be patient and listen to that little voice. If you listen, it will guide you exactly where you are required to go. Oh yeah and let go of all expectations of how it shows up because sometimes the picture is created by the mind; however, the heart knows the truth of what is required. It is an interesting tangle to navigate. Just trust in the heart is the key.

Looking back over my life now, it is so interesting to observe the threads created, patterns repeated, and lessons to grow from. Acceptance of myself is at the top of the list of hurdles I jumped over and over again. Growing up, I always felt like an outcast, never belonging anywhere that I drummed to a different tune yet did my best to be in tune with everyone else. It took me all this time to realize that I had been fighting against myself and took it out on the rest of the world around me. Blaming everyone else for my pain and not seeing that I was creating it all myself. I could not see myself. I could not accept the person I was and how I viewed the world and see it through my lens. I remember all the times I could not speak up and express myself, for who would want to hear my thoughts? This way of being kept me from my voice and truth. Yet there was a part of me that had no problem fighting for others and speaking my mind when required. I did everything I could to keep control of this part of me until I decided to let go, and all began to unravel. Letting go of this control has opened me up to learning to speak my truth, what I desire and knowing it is safe to express this. Knowing it is ok if someone has a different view than you. Accepting this is how I like to be in the world, and I don't have to hide anymore. It has empowered me to not allow the thought of others' judgments to stop me from my goals and what I desire to do. Now, to be honest, I still have those old programs that run through my head, and I go into doubt and question myself; however, now I have the tools to tell myself that is not the truth and change the narrative. This, in turn, brings me so much joy that I am opening to honor me.

Another huge hurdle that I moved through is learning boundaries and discerning others' intentions and actions. This one lesson I did not want to face which left me with a physical reminder to stand up for myself and it is ok to say no. I feel this is a huge one for a lot of people out in the world today. I allowed people in my world to take advantage of my kindness and went against myself to make them happy until it left me scared. So now I have a constant reminder to face the truth and set boundaries with others, learn to discern that if something doesn't feel right, step back and evaluate before embracing, being silent is a strength, and choosing peace over chaos. I have learned there are different flavors out in the world, and you just have to taste and find your favorite flavor. Doesn't mean you can't have a taste of others just remember it is just a taste, not a full cone. It's if people in your world melt away that don't co-create with you. It's okay to say no if it does not bring you joy. It's okay to express how people make you feel, be open and honest, and know they might not be able to receive it. And it's okay to be okay with others not understanding where you are coming from because you know you are at peace and joy around your actions, and that's all that matters. Standing tall in being the love you are, and it is your choice on who and what you choose to interact and take action within your life. The golden nugget here is to allow yourself to be the clarity in the chaos, stay aligned with you, and engage only when required. For in the clarity of who you are is the strength to move thru any situation with the utmost grace. Staying in that alignment is what we must strive to master.

Forgetness is another wisdom key I have picked up along the way to assist in my navigating this new dream I am creating. Now, forgetness and forgive-ness are two words that dance together like precise strands of DNA intertwining to create. You see when we can learn to forget the emotional trigger someone has cast upon us then we can open to forgive. I have found in my life and listening to others' stories there is a key shift of living in the past. This is by learning that what was put upon us, that person was doing the best they could at that moment no matter what the situation. Now, I know that this opens a can of worms for so many points of view; however, still, no matter what stems from that truth, from my point of view. The story will always be the story the inner trigger is the healing obstacle to tackle and detach from. For in that, detachment is the key to freedom of the soul. Once you have that you can forgive for it is only a story, not a quantum entanglement stuck in your field. So, when one can forget that emotional feeling, then one can forgive from the heart and take back their power. That's what's so funny: when we hold on to things, we are giving our power to whatever that is. When we open to release that, we claim ourselves back and can forgive. At 50, this was huge and clear to look at. If you travel down this road, just always remember to be kind to yourself during the process of healing 50 years of heartache and pain that take time to completely release. Then, one day, you wake up, and someone will trigger you; however, that emotional stir in the pit of your stomach is not there. That's the day you are free, and it feels amazing. I always remember during my aunt's transition to the other side, she lifted her hands up and said NO MORE, NO MORE, and I knew that was the moment she surrendered to death—a very powerful moment to witness and a reminder that is how simple it really can be.

Embrace 50 and beyond because this is really the time in your life to truly grow into you. The YOU without all the baggage that you were carrying. It is a freeing and a new sense of flowing that I am learning to walk in these shoes of a new dream for me. I am finally able to embrace many things that I have held in fear of being judged. The crusty layers have fallen off, and there is a new light in my heart. A softening of my soul in that I am finally able to see where I was living from a place of survival and embracing truly living. This new level of gratitude and appreciation is opening in my heart as I move forward to dance with life. It has been a journey, and looking back, I would not change a thing. For it has brought me here in my 50s, and I have traveled a full road of experiences, and now I give myself permission to play in the light of me. Laugh and enjoy the beautiful world we live in amongst the chaos. I have gratitude in my heart for this gift I am able to experience, which is being human.

So, dance in the dream of love and spiral to create a life that brings joy in your heart. Live that life, and don't look back.

21

About Rebecka Gregory

Rebecka Gregory CHt embracing the light she truly is and sharing her gifts and knowledge planting the seeds for others to find theirs. Rebecka's journey led her on a path to study many modalities in the energy, shamanic, and cosmic world. Her knowledge experience remembrance path began with learning about the Toltec teachings and led her to learn the art of Hypnotherapy. Along the way diving into different energy modalities, shamanic practices, plant medicine, traveling to sacred sites, and the honor of working with some amazing teachers. The cosmic truth of her heart song opened when she received the art of vibrational resonance. Giving herself the gift of saying YES to digging deep into the darkness of herself was priceless…. A gift that she has realized is the key to it all… Loving YOU and living in love. And learning to BE. She was co-host of the Cosmic Insight podcast.

Website: www.rebeckagregory.com

Chapter Three

If You're Ready to Face Some Truths, 50 Might Just Be What You Were Waiting For...

by Dr. Johanneke Kodde

I am nearly 50, and I feel fabulous.

It wasn't always this way, and it may change again in the future.

But I'm claiming it.

Maybe I'm lucky, maybe I have good 'genes' (although my mother collapsed with anemia due to years of heavy bleeding), or maybe I'm privileged. Still, I'm also a medical professional who has seen hundreds of women go through midlife with a wide spectrum of experiences, and I am good at seeing patterns. And I am a human who has gone through her own shit and upheaval in the past three or so years. I sometimes say my middle name is 'self-development' because I am insatiably curious about human behavior (including my own) so you could say I am a psychologist and an intuitive disguised as a doctor.

We don't have a body so we can suffer. We don't get symptoms and diseases to make our lives miserable. Our body is an extremely sensitive, fine-tuned, and complex system that is in continuous exchange with its environment. And we co-create our reality with our

23

body, mind, and soul. Our souls inhabit a human body in order to experience life. And all that comes with that. Through life, our souls can learn, play, and evolve. Our amazing mind has the capacity to observe and be actively involved in all that is happening in our body. But this takes awareness and practice.

We need awareness of our thoughts, emotions, beliefs, and feelings. Bringing subconscious desires, programs, and inherited behaviors to our conscious awareness so that we can influence and upgrade them. If we can do this, we become the driver rather than a passenger; we take care of our vehicle to get the best ride. We will be more inclined to clean our windows so we can see the beauty this earth has to offer. We are more likely to check on our engine and take action if something needs attention.

But of course, our bodies are infinitely more complex and receptive than a car. Every cell has its own intelligence; every bacteria has its own purpose to fulfill. Every thought we think has an impact, creates a cascade of emotions, and with that, chemical, electrical, and vibrational messages bounce around our system. Every person we are in close contact with influences our energy, and loved ones can have an influence that shows that space and time are just constructs within our 3D reality.

What makes me say all this, which you may call philosophical talk? How does this apply to your life and your hot flashes, sleepless nights, and creaky joints? Or, maybe you have become more anxious and self-conscious in your 40s, even though you have not really felt like this since your teens? Or you get moments of rage, where you barely recognize yourself when you shout and swear at anyone who happens to be in your vicinity (most likely your significant other or children). Or have palpitations, panic attacks, and are no longer interested in sex. You can't do it anymore, juggling a million and one things, a job, a family, pets, elderly parents, and dinner parties, and have completely lost the motivation or energy to do the exercise that is supposed to keep you healthy. You are too tired to go to a farmer's market and prepare 'healthy' food for yourself, let alone for anyone else. Maybe you are still doing all of this for others but have not taken time for yourself for years, or the only way to unwind is with that large glass of wine (or two) and a G&T with friends occasionally. Only to need more coffee to get you through the next day.

Any of this sound familiar? You are not alone. I have been there, and most women in their 40s and 50s are there. But it doesn't need to be this way. There is so much wisdom in our bodies and the messages it is trying to give. There is so much silver that can be polished and gold that can be mined in your own life. So much joy and creativity you may be missing out on.

So where to start?

I suggest you start by stopping to do, do, do. Do all the things for all the people. Try a different pace, get quiet, take a break, and stare out of the window. Start by getting curious and letting uncomfortable feelings and truths bubble up from your deepest depths. In order to allow time and space for this, you will need to become more discerning. To start saying no when something feels wrong or off, or you are tired. To become more selective in your relationships and kinder to yourself. To really prioritize yourself, not by a token bath or massage (although these can be very nourishing, of course) but by getting to know your desires, your feelings, your personal unique way of tuning into your body's wisdom and your intuition. And this is difficult to do with depleted adrenals. This is difficult when you see symptoms as inconveniences to get rid of. You may well be feeling bone tired, so it is scary to slow down or stop. But the risk is worth taking because you cannot escape yourself. If you keep running, you will trip, sooner or later, with increasingly severe consequences.

This is why this time in life, the (peri)menopause is SO valuable and amazing if you are prepared to see that it is happening FOR you, not against you. You may want to use medication like HRT to feel a little better, but it can never replace the opportunity to listen to your soul and understand yourself more deeply. To course-correct if the path you are galloping down isn't quite the right one. To reduce the demands others place on you and the expectations you place on yourself. Your hormones are changing for a reason. Because your role is changing with your increasing life experience and wisdom. Less estrogen means less inclination to please everyone. Less energy to spin all the plates. Less patience with bullshit and so-called cultural obligations and expectations. Time to move out of the 'mothering' phase, when you either have children or you look after projects, pets or other people, or all of those combined. Time to move into and embrace the WILD WOMAN, akin to the energy of autumn- shedding, letting go, evaluating, correcting. The wild woman needs to break with old patterns and shed the conditioning and programming she has been imprinted with as a child and was given to her parents by many generations of ancestors. This is no mean feat, and if we suppress this inner transformative energy, we risk repeating patriarchal ideas in new guises. If we use hormonal treatments to 'be ourselves again' and stay youthful, we are actually falling into a trap that is so insidious that many powerful and influential women are not even aware they are caught in it.

Let me explain. As I see it, a lot of female empowerment still serves the patriarchy, and female freedom fighters are still shouting from a place of either victimhood or old paradigm masculine values. Take the contraceptive pill that is still given to many teenage girls to help with their (sometimes painful) bleeds, their skin or to make sure they can 'fit in' with school standards or societal expectations.

Of course, the hormonal contraceptive pill was necessary for the participation and validation of women in the workplace and gave them tremendous newfound freedom, but it has ended up creating a monster made of unattainable masculine standards to push through, spin an impossible number of plates and feel weak for showing too much emotion.

In the same way, HRT provides a reprieve from debilitating sleepless nights and the ability to keep up the highly estrogenized standards that we have set for ourselves. But we use it with a high risk of perpetuating the myth of the everlasting summer, continuing to be at the service of all and sundry.

I get it; heavy, painful periods are annoying. And they make us stop and turn inwards. We owe it to our daughters, all teenage girls, and indeed all women to wake up to our complicity in maintaining systems that are designed for a homogeneous mass of competitive people-pleasers who are told to 'get on with it' and 'push through.' Schools, sports environments, and workplaces still largely lack the flexibility that a fully embodied human needs. Women have many fresh ideas at the start of their cycle (like spring) when they come out of their inward intuitive menstrual phase. This energy builds to a creative, proactive practical (summer) phase of planning and executing when they are more energized and outward facing. A time of action and excitement then is followed by an evaluation, a slowing, a natural pulling back of energy (like autumn), masterfully guided by estrogen reducing and progesterone increasing. This is often experienced as unbearable when the critic can bring up anger, resentment, a realization of boundaries having been trampled, and a re-balancing of the state of play.

However, if this could be seen as a valuable and essential time in which we can learn and grow whilst leaning into how clearly our nature is part of all nature, it becomes a superb tool, leading us beautifully into a time of stillness, for an internal reset, when our bleed sets in (inner winter).

Hormonal contraception suppresses this beautiful dance of our moods and energies. It often completely stops our own cycle in favor of a simplistic tune. Very practical. Very handy for exams, swimming galas, or school trips. Immensely helpful for stressed out (peri-menopausal) mothers in loggerheads with their unreasonable daughters.

Allowing women to have a natural cycle will help infuse our world with much-needed feminine ways of leadership, which are based on inclusion, intuition, and collaboration. Of course, this requires women to take responsibility and become clued up and vocal about their own energy and moods. The last thing we need is a world solely steered by mood swings and going with the 'flow' at all times.

However, it is also time we ditch the admiration of busyness, goals, and action as the only way to achieve. We don't need a matriarchy, nor a patriarchy; we need a world that balances determination, focus, and activity with receptivity, creativity, flow, and interconnectedness with nature, seasons, and cycles. It can never be either or. It can only be both, in an eternal dance and embrace, in full service and admiration of each other.

The reality is that we are still, mostly, deeply conditioned by the masculine way. This is not to say any man is directly responsible or to blame for this. I am talking about thousands of years of imprinting by organized religion, industrialization, colonization and scientific developments. Logic has ruled over intuition. And it has brought us many advances. But it is too limiting, and our system is designed to bring as many people as possible in line, but this takes away their uniqueness and creativity. An example that is happening and causing widespread fallout of our systems is neurodiversity. These children cannot and will not be conditioned to follow the rules. The accumulation of all of their needs is creating a perfect storm that is breaking the old-school ways, and more and more neurodiverse adults are reinventing themselves in innovative ways of working, which shows us the rigidity of the workplace and is breaking the mold to allow flexibility.

These are exciting times because, due to technology like the internet and smartphones, anyone can see what is going on and going down on this planet; oppression and destruction can no longer be hidden, and there is no other way left than to address it. The tables are turning and this time we need to have four different strong legs to keep it upright. Two legs with masculine and two legs with feminine energy. Each represents an element- Air, Fire, Water, and Earth. Four legs for the four seasons. So humanity can start to move in an upward spiral, always changing, evaluating, and renewing with loving intention.

For an actual revolution of our consciousness, we need every single person to find their unique talents and gifts so we can work together and collaborate with mutual respect and understanding rather than be dominated by governmental and religious leaders and large corporations. The systems are no longer fit for purpose; they cannot protect and provide for us. We need to find our own truth and strength so that we can contribute in a resourceful and personal way.

This is where the power of the menopause transition comes to the fore. In my observation at all ages in different ways, we are given the opportunity to upgrade our own systems. If we get a bit too caught up in day-to-day activities, our body will remind us to pay attention. It will literally make us stop with a viral illness, an injury, or worse. If we pop a pill or refuse to slow down, it will up the antics and something more noticeable will come along. A chronic illness may develop if we ignore the messages as we accumulate unprocessed emotions and repeat generational programs. Auto-immune conditions are a prime example of this. Remember, auto-immune means that our immune system is fighting against itself. What stronger message can we get? And even cancer is a representation of an imbalance in our immune regulation. Natural cell death is not working properly, and some cells get overactive, over-reproduce, and over-consume. Sounds a bit like the human population on planet Earth if you ask me.

Unfortunately, what we are meant to believe is that we need to fight AGAINST these diseases. We are victims, and the only way out is to try harder to struggle against it. Try to beat it. Beat what? Ourselves? That is like fighting against war with more violence, against poverty with more inequality, and using dominance and suppression, control and submission. Sounds like the patriarchy all over again.

So back to you, struggling with your menopause and the shit that is being thrown up in its wake. No, it isn't pleasant or pretty sometimes. Yes, it is FOR you and so necessary. Let's take a closer look at some of the symptoms I mentioned earlier.

Hot flashes- your body temperature is going all over the place. The direct physiological reason is the hormonal changes, for sure.

Although interestingly, not everyone gets them. Let's look at them metaphorically, which is much more fun and illuminating. What if this heat is there to burn away all that doesn't suit and doesn't serve you anymore? Ever heard of a phoenix? It burns to the ground in a mighty fire, to be reborn from the ashes. You don't need to sacrifice everything and everyone in some massive bonfire 'release' ceremony, but I bet you some things you are holding onto really aren't worth it. Get curious. Make some changes. If you don't do it now, it will happen in another, possibly more destructive way further down the road.

What about mood swings, including anger and sadness? What if you are literally no longer able to tolerate what you previously thought was acceptable? Being the jack of all trades, being the provider, people pleaser, juggler extraordinaire. What if you are harboring (often barely conscious) resentments, regrets, and what-ifs? That parent that never saw you or expected too much, the work colleague from whom you tolerated their dominant or hurtful behavior, the partner with whom you are bouncing projections and expectations backwards and forwards without fully expressing them in a healthy way. Well, now it all comes out unfiltered. Raw anger and rage lead to blame, guilt, and counter-blame. Rage turned inwards can lead to inflammation or depression. Not a pretty picture. So let it out but lose the guilt and blame. There is no blame in any of this. It's merely dynamics playing out, having played out for years with nowhere to go. Release them, sit with them, and go to those memories until you find the gold within. And if it is too much to do alone, find a therapist, talk to a friend, or join a group or circle.

Another example: lack of energy, fatigue, and lack of motivation. Of course, make sure you get some blood tests done, and if you have deficiencies, anemia, or otherwise, get this treated. But even so-called 'real' medical issues are merely outcomes of ignoring your body's messages until they become more obvious. A lack of energy is always, in some way, related to the balance of action and rest, activity and restoration, stress, and nervous system regulation. Animals cannot help themselves but to have a nap after spending precious energy on finding food, mating, or building a nest, and or shaking off tension after a stressful encounter. However, human animals have this clever brain, which has, somewhere down the evolutionary path, been given superhero status. So it can ignore or overrule almost anything the body is communicating until it can't. And then we'll know about it. Burnout. Chronic fatigue. Post-viral fatigue. Brain fog. And then we feel cheated because we have lost our ability to push through. What if we should have stopped months or years ago? Our adrenals are so done with pumping out cortisol chronically that it is adding to the problems of hormonal imbalance, blood sugar regulation, and many other regulatory systems. We are not meant to keep going regardless or because we have the willpower to do so. Sooner or later there will be a day when we can no longer do this. And if lack of motivation is your first sign, take it. Listen to it. Stop the willpower show. You will not regret it.

I can write a whole book about all the different possible symptoms, but I hope you get the idea by now.

Circling back to where I started, I have had my share of shit going down in my forties. You can read all about it in the book Lessons Learned the Hard Way, chapter 19. But I learned to listen. I stopped and rested. I had coaching, went to transformative retreats, and took a hard look at all the societal, parental, and ancestral patterns that were playing out in my life, my relationship, and my parenting style. I made changes. I quit my hard-earned, prestigious medical job to become an entrepreneur. I followed my inner calling and course corrected. Lucky for him, I did not ditch my husband; we keep reinventing our partnership. I prioritize friendships that bring me joy and fill me up. I go into nature a lot. I have embraced my (unpredictable) cycle. I only exercise when I have enough energy. I travel and spend time with people and in places that elevate me. And I am on a mission to spread the word about the importance of embracing the transformative power of the menopause far and wide…

About Johanneke Kodde

Dr Johanneke Kodde is an experienced family doctor, who believes that the awareness and integration of body, mind and soul will help many people to better understand their symptoms, face mental health challenges and uncover and follow their hidden desires and passions. She is also a coach, speaker and wildly wise woman.

www.bodymindsouldoctor.com

Instagram: @bodymindsouldoctor

Facebook: Body Mind Soul Doctor (business) and Johanneke Kodde (personal)

LinkedIn: Dr Johanneke Kodde

Chapter Four

Lulus & Muumuus: My Journey from Beauty to Beast & Back

by Denise Nussbaum, Ph.D.

It was my wedding day. March 21, 1997. The Celestial Equinox. A time for embracing balance and renewal. A moment of equilibrium. It was also the day my new husband revealed to me that he had another identity.

Scene: My wedding night. Following the age-old ritual of presenting myself to my new husband for the consummation of our marriage, I emerged from the dressing room in my beautiful new negligee. I was feeling fantastic, so confident, so good about myself and my sexuality that I actually raised my arms in the air and exclaimed, "tadaaaaah!"

He was thrilled. (Yay!) You might even say delighted (Woot!). He walked toward me with his arms outstretched. This was the moment … just like in the movies. Was this a dream? Have I finally found my person? Will I finally be the wife and mother I am destined to be? He placed his hands on my shoulders and spun me around (how romantic!) and looked at the tag (huh?).

His next words were, "Do you think they make this in my size?". (Wah waaaah.)

After my shiny new spouse revealed to me that he was a crossdresser -- once I wrapped my head around it -- I tried to understand, to accommodate, and to accept it. I had just said my marriage vows. For better or for worse. After all, I was a sociology professor and taught gender studies. If anyone understood gender fluidity, it was me.

In the end, while I applauded his choice to live his truth, I could not embrace his behavior as my husband. It didn't fit into my internalized idea of what a husband should be, i.e., masculine. Looking back on my girlhood dreams of love and marriage, Prince Charming was definitely not wearing a wig and size 14 stilettos. Not surprisingly, it didn't help that once he told me, he quit his job and sat around in drag all day watching hermaphrodite porn. Our marriage ended after one year.

Gender fluidity. What is gender? Why is it important? How do we learn it? Why are we so deeply rooted in society's expectations of how we should act, what we should wear, and who we should love? Why do we love who we love? Why do we hate our bodies? Why do we find it so difficult to love and accept ourselves? Why don't we feel like we're good enough? Pretty enough? Smart enough? Nice enough? Accommodating enough? Why do we find inner peace so elusive? Why do we torture ourselves trying to live up to what we know are unrealistic expectations of our feelings, appearances, and behavior? Especially as we age? Shouldn't we know better by now?

Learning How to Be Me

I was a child of the sixties. The Vietnam War was raging, the civil rights movement was erupting and becoming increasingly violent, and the sexual revolution was intensifying. There was never any discussion of war or civil rights in my suburban, middle-class neighborhood. Granted, these topics were easy to avoid back then, as the networks only broadcast 30 minutes of news a day, and my parents didn't discuss current events. They and their friends were apolitical and seemingly uninterested in the world around them.

What a great privilege it was to live in a place (both mentally and physically) unaffected by inequalities, oppression, and war. We lived blissfully unaware of the political and social turmoil that lurked in nearby cities and abroad. However, the sexual revolution was not only acknowledged in my household, but it was also given a seat at the table. "Free Love" was welcomed with open arms. It entered amidst great applause down a red shag carpet, through our front door, and sat its happy, naked ass down on our red velvet, plastic-covered sofa.

As young children, my brother and I watched a lot of television. We were basically raised by the "idiot box." We watched cartoons before school and on Saturday mornings and sitcoms at night. We were immersed in tales of happy families, heroes, and dreams of happily ever after. Seemingly harmless, right? What could go wrong? Little did we know, we were being taught how to live, what to think, how to act. TV taught us who is good and who is evil. Perhaps most significantly for a girl teetering on the edge of adolescence, the "boob tube" revealed to us what was beautiful and why it was so important. It taught us what we could do and who we could be, what was possible, and what was unattainable. Media taught us who to love and who to hate. Even if that hate was turned inward.

What lessons could young people possibly learn from cartoons? From Mighty Mouse, I learned that no matter what trouble lurked for Sweet Polly Purebred, her hero would save her. If the message was unclear, he literally sang it a cappella as he flew to rescue Polly from the bad guys, "Here I come to save the daaaaay … !" With a little help from the pill in his bracelet (missed opportunity by Big Pharma for product placement) he could vanquish any bad guy and save the helpless female. Lessons: pills are good; women are constantly in need of rescue; your hero will save you. Right after Mighty Mouse we watched Dudley Do-Right rescue Nelle from the railroad tracks, time and again. Of course, the blond-haired, blue-eyed Canadian Mountie bested the evil dark, and smarmy Boris and Natasha every time. Lessons: the damsel in distress gets her man; even evil women must be beautiful with long hair, big boobs, and a 12-inch waist; Russia is bad. On Saturdays, we watched Popeye and witnessed two men

35

fighting over an anorexic, fragile, helpless female who has no voice of her own. Who will win the competition for Olive Oil? Lessons: you are valuable if men fight over you; startlingly skinny is desirable; women do not choose their man, they are chosen.

Our "education" continued as we watched Disney movies. Snow White cooks and cleans for the dwarves as she waits for her Prince Charming; Ariel gives up her voice in order to win her man with her body; Belle changes the violent and abusive Beast with love, forgiveness, and submission. Lessons: serve and submit; do anything to get your man; you can change him if you just love him enough. Of all the lessons we learn from cartoons, this is one of the most dangerous. The normalization of intimate partner violence (IPV) and abuse is a dangerous road to travel. Overall, roughly ¼ of individuals have perpetrated IPV, with rates among younger dating populations on the rise. Statistics surrounding emotional abuse and control reveal that a staggering 80% of individuals have committed emotional abuse. The consequences include higher rates of psychological symptoms and disorders and increased probability of depression, anxiety, post-traumatic stress disorder (PTSD), and substance abuse.

Still today, cartoons represent female characters in a twisted, exaggerated version of femininity. The characters have highly sexualized bodies and often a coy seductiveness. In the end, love and happily ever after come true once her hero arrives for the rescue. The lessons don't stop at gender. We have seen Latinos portrayed as lazy Chihuahuas, African Americans portrayed as human-wannabe orangutans and gang members, Arabs as barbarians, Jews as money-hungry shysters, Asians as treacherous, manipulative Siamese Cats, and Native Americans as wild savages. All of us are stereotyped, wrapped up in neat and tidy little packages. Ready for judgment.

Our instruction did not always come in animated form. The Wizard of Oz was a favorite of mine. I could always relate to Dorothy. A naïve, simple girl from a small town. Resilient and determined to find her way home. Originally a depression-era allegory of poverty, famine, and industrialization, the movie has undergone many iterations; however, the themes remain the same. The Yellow Brick Road symbolizes hope and the path to happiness and fulfillment. We learn your life may seem dull and colorless (the film was in black and white until they stepped foot on the yellow brick road), but if you are good and innocent (Dorothy), work hard (schlep down the yellow brick road) and face your challenges (flying monkeys and evil witches) bravely, intelligently and compassionately (cowardly lion, scarecrow, tin man) you will find your way back home, your happily ever after … which just happens to be where you began, home with your family and your person. Tidy.

By the time I was eleven years old, I knew what I needed to do: be beautiful, kind, sweet, accommodating, resilient, and patient, so my person would find me and sweep me off my feet. Just follow the yellow brick road …

Later on, we watched Ellie Mae use her body to get what she wanted in The Beverly Hillbillies, despite her obvious intellectual limitations. We learned about beauty and dating from The Brady Bunch ("Marcia, Marcia, Marcia!") and The Partridge Family. I learned from Laugh-In that I was already too fat to be pretty, thanks to Twiggy and Goldie Hawn. However, as the second wave of feminism reared her beautiful, majestic head, hope entered the "curriculum." I was drawn to shows that seemed to resist traditional representations of weak women and strong men. In The Dick Van Dyke Show, Laura Petrie strives to be the perfect wife and mother amidst many discussions about the role of women in the home and in the workforce. In the final season, we see Laura wearing slacks, a bold feminist statement for the sixties. Even The Munsters and The Addams Family embraced strong matriarchs who wielded power in the family.

Subsequently, That Girl and The Mary Tyler Moore Show broke ground with a protagonist who was a single, working woman, not just the wife, girlfriend, or widow of a male counterpart. Mary Tyler Moore revolved around Mary Richards, a single career woman in her thirties, who had been dumped by her fiancé. This show explored the complexity of the female characters and actually produced two spin-offs, Rhoda and Phyllis, also starring strong independent women. Perhaps my favorite show was Bewitched. Samantha was just a housewife, but she had more power than her husband, albeit from witchcraft. Who was splitting hairs?

Another show I found empowering in the 1970s was Charlie's Angels. Yes, the female crime-fighting crew was controlled by males … and yes, they were all hot and sexualized. However… Did you see the one where Farrah chased down the bad guys on a skateboard, not a strand of her perfectly feathered hair out of place? Come on! Perfection! Goals.

As I grew older, I paid more and more attention to advertisements as I fulfilled my all-American role as a good little consumer. It turned out that I was consuming more than the products being sold. Ads are influential because they have very little time and space to get their messages across, so symbolism is significant. Both males and females are regularly shown in highly stereotypical poses. Female hands are weak as they cradle, caress, and delicately trace the outline of the product being sold. Conversely, male hands are powerful, assertive, and controlling; they grasp the product firmly. Similarly, men are shown in upright positions gazing directly at the viewer, again, powerful, engaged, and in control. Women, on the other hand, are often shown lying down, vulnerable, or off-balance, often with a coy knee-bend or a flirtatious head tilt, or their fingers in and around their mouths. Their gaze looks away from the viewer, inattentive … exposed. All of these messages reflect age-old representations of women as submissive, powerless, and sexually available, while men are dominant, powerful, and in control.

Why do these representations matter, and how do they affect us? These images reproduce and glamorize images of women as weak and vulnerable in victim-ready poses. Self-defense classes stress the opposite: control of one's body and one's safety requires being alert and aware of your surroundings. Studies of violent men reveal they often choose their victims based on body posture and non-verbal cues.

The 1970s was a great decade for music. I spent much of my childhood alone in my bedroom, listening to LPs and reading the record jackets (a lost art form, if you ask me). I also listened to AM radio and mentally downloaded each and every song. The music I grew up with, the music of the 1970s, is literally the soundtrack to my life, as I'm sure is true for many of us. Music affects us deeply, both emotionally and psychologically. The lyrics, tone, and tempo of each song each tell a separate story. Popular songs are repeated over and over again, and their messages -- both obvious and subtle, overt and subliminal -- saturate our consciousness.

In the music of the early 1970s, love was more idealized, and sex wasn't necessarily the goal. These folks were singing about romance and true love. Diana Ross promised there "Ain't no mountain high enough," and Michael Jackson swore, "I'll Be There." Even sweet Donny Osmond insisted, "Go Away Little Girl," because he wanted to remain faithful to his one true love. Later in the decade, we heard more and more about the pitfalls of love. Paul Simon would teach us "Fifty Ways to Leave Your Lover," while Mary MacGregor was "Torn Between Two Lovers," and Thelma Houston begged, "Don't Leave Me This Way." As the decade comes to a close, Barbara Streisand laments, "You Don't Bring Me Flowers," the Doobies warn us about "What a Fool Believes," and Gloria Gaynor proudly proclaims, "I Will Survive". As an adolescent girl, these messages stuck with me. Love is complicated, but I will survive. How bad could it be?

Feminism was quick to join the party with Helen Reddy's "I Am Woman" and Carly Simon's "You're So Vain." Who can forget Linda Ronstadt's "You're No Good"? I truly connected with these amazing women and saw myself as a strong girl who could make it on her own without the help of a man – they couldn't be trusted. But then again, John Travolta promised, "You're the One That I Want," Peaches and Herb were "Reunited," and Exile wanted to "Kiss You All Over," so who am I to knock a good thing? Increasingly, music became more overtly sexualized with artists like Marvin Gaye's "Let's Get It On," KC and the Sunshine Band's "That's the Way (I Like It)", and Rod Stewart's "Do You Think I'm Sexy?" My earliest memory of combining music and sexuality was the Steve Miller song "The Joker." When he sang, "You're the cutest thing that I ever did see/I really love your peaches, wanna shake your tree …," I was still young and naive, but even I knew he wasn't singing about the fall harvest. And finally, messages about civil rights also crept into 1970s pop music with Cher's "Half Breed," The Hues Corporation's "Rock the Boat," and Eric Clapton's "I Shot the Sheriff". Armed with these teachings, I set off to experience becoming a woman and finding my person. Follow the yellow brick road …

Whiskers, Sisters, and Too Many Misters

When I realized my body represented power and danger, I was fourteen years old. My best friend's drunk father pulled me down to sit on his lap at a pool party. He and his equally intoxicated friends laughed and made comments while I sat there, bewildered by their attention. I remember a feeling of discomfort and shame, but I didn't acknowledge that. What I remembered most was the attention. I liked it. I was innocent and had no idea as to the implications of what was happening. It would be years until I put it all together. Years before I realized I had blindly, but willingly, entered the female role of object, subordinate, and pleaser. I was now the accommodator of the male gaze, touch, and control. I would occupy this role for over forty years.

Once I had the taste of power, I became a junkie. After all, there was nothing wrong with sex and sexuality, it was the '70s, right? Feminism was alive and well, and the world was changing. I dated a lot in those days with little regard for my "reputation". I would soon learn that the whole free love thing really only benefitted males and that the sexual revolution didn't actually apply to women. While promiscuous males were called "studs," we women were still "sluts". Case in point: In the summer of 1987, I was backpacking alone through Europe. While traveling through Italy, I fell asleep all alone in a train compartment and awoke to a strange man trying to stick his big toe inside my shorts and panties. I jumped up screaming and kicking, and soon, a male train employee came running in and told the man to leave. When I asked the man, in Italian, what they were going to do to the man who had accosted me, he answered in English, "Leave him alone, American slut."

The world hasn't changed much, but I have. Even as mature women, we are still subjected to sexualized scrutiny. When I was young, I was referred to as "hot," meaning men wanted to have sex with me. In my 30s, I was referred to as a MILF, (mother I'd like to f*ck). Okay, tacky, but hey, I'm still desirable. In my 40s, I was a "cougar". Now I'm a GILF (grandmother I'd like to f*ck) and apparently someone who used to be good-looking. True story: Just last week, Larry, the repairman, was at our home fixing some screens. Larry is in his 70s and has been doing work for us for years. On this trip, Larry noticed a painting of me and my husband on our wedding day, 15 years ago. Larry stopped in front of the painting, looked at it, and exclaimed, "Ma'am, I'm not saying you're not nice lookin' now, but you were a real looker back in the day!" Fuck you, Larry! Ok, probably not the most civilized response, but WHAT IS the appropriate response to a comment like that? As women, we're supposed to smile and accept the "compliment." I stand by my response. I am looking forward to my 60s and 70s when I will no doubt be referred to as a "handsome woman".

But Larry was right; this old girl ain't what she used to be. But SO WHAT?! Today, my body is not winning any swimsuit model competitions or bringing any "milkshakes to the yard" (sorry, Kelis). Nope. Collagen has left the building to make space for cellulite, melting skin and hair in all the wrong places. Wearing Lulus (Lululemon yoga pants) has given way to wearing MuuMuus that better accommodate my ever-expanding waistline and my ever-present hot flashes. At 59 years old, my body serves me like a beloved old truck. She has a few dings and dents, but she gets me where I'm going. True, I always need to warm her up before I put her in drive, and yes, sometimes I ask, "Is she going to start today?" She could use a new paint job and probably an engine haul-over, but I appreciate her loyalty and her efficiency. And best of all, I'm no longer a victim of my gender role. I am exactly who I want to be when I want to be her ... for the most part. The best part is that I finally

41

found my person: It's me! But I could not have arrived here without my tribe of women.

Friendships over 50 are special, much more intimate, and real. Gone is the cattiness, judgment, and competition of youthful friendships. We now collectively understand we were duped and we remind each other often. We realized the lure of sexual promiscuity, the promises of happily ever after, the myths about true love, and the distortions about beauty and the body were all lies. But that's okay. We survived. Yes, our bodies have "matured" along with our minds. At my age, peeing myself is no longer a catastrophe ... really, it's high praise for the person who made me laugh ... like slurping noodles in Japan. One person's faux pas is another's measure of a good time. When I was younger, we laughed until tears ran down our cheeks. Today, we laugh until the tears run down our legs. But shit, at least we're still laughing.

About Dr. Denise Nussbaum

After backpacking around the world on a ten-dollar-a-day budget for the better part of three years, Dr. Nussbaum earned her Ph.D. in sociology in 1999. Applying her education to her life experience, she became a Professor and Department Chair at Mt. San Jacinto College for 22 years, teaching and mentoring 100s of students to think critically about the world around them. During this time, Dr. Nussbaum published several articles and book chapters in the areas of prejudice, discrimination, and social inequalities. In 2003, she was honored by the Academic Senate for California Community Colleges with the prestigious Stanback-Stroud Diversity Award. Today, Dr. Nussbaum is retired from academia but still writes about the effects of social institutions on our social identities and our everyday lives.

Chapter Five
Are You Ready to Die?
by Shelley Whizin

"The fear of death follows from the fear of life.

A man who lives fully is prepared to die at any time." – Mark Twain

It was 1986, and my first trip to Peru on a Journey of Initiation with Dr. Alberto Villoldo, then Professor at San Francisco State University, and Don Eduardo Calderon, the Peruvian shaman who had a vision that he must teach the art of shamanism to the Western world, otherwise shamanism would become a lost art.

I was in the second group of human potential workers, healers, artists, and psychologists that Alberto took to Peru, investigating how energy medicine and visualization could change the chemistry in the brain. We were to re-enact ancient Ayahuasca and San Pedro ceremonies at the power centers in Peru, studying the ancient wisdom teachings of the Indian Medicine Wheel. Each direction of the wheel was infused with purposeful meaning, and life-altering perspectives, symbolized by a power animal with specific characteristics and qualities.

Starting in the South, which was represented by the snake, we found ourselves in the Nazca Plains, where the mysterious carvings etched into the ground for thousands of years had no sign of footprints. It's still a mystery today. You can only see these carvings from the air. We flew over these carvings in small 2-seat airplanes that were put together with spit, glue, and rubber bands. I felt like I was in an Indiana Jones movie. This was an awesome adventure!

The snake represented the shedding of one's skin, letting go of all archetypes, stereotypes, and ancestral history, preparing us to be fully present for the West. We each walked along the path of the great spiral, (representing the snake), holding onto a staff in our right hand, determined not to be pulled off our path from the ancient spirits that resided there.

As witnesses, we held the space for each other to walk, while observing the spirits appear from beneath the spiral, pulling each person's energy to step off the path. We had to be steadfast in our quest to make it to the end. As a group, we became the guardians, holding the space for each one to make it through. We then picked a place for a vision quest, sat in silence, at one with the universe, quiet in our destination.

As I sat looking up at the endless night sky, I could feel the earth beneath me sending its pulsating life force through my body, and to my surprise, I experienced a natural orgasm that shot through me like something I had never experienced in my life. "WOW," I thought. "I was one with mother earth and father sky." Something in me awakened that would last a lifetime.

Two days later, destined for Machu Picchu we traveled clockwise to the power of the West, represented by the rainbow jaguar, serving as the bridge between the physical and spiritual worlds.

Because Alberto was part of the Department of Anthropology and connected with the government of Peru, when all the tourists had gone home, we were privileged to conduct our all-night ceremonies. We gathered around Spirit Flight Rock, where each person was told to lay down, one by one.

According to the shaman, the job of every human is to go out in cohesive light through the heart, where all energies converge and leave the body. It was my turn to lay on Spirit Flight Rock. The silence of the universe was deafening, and the stillness of the stars was as if no time and space existed. And then, the silence stopped, and I heard a voice.

"Are you ready to die?" the shaman asked.

I heard myself thinking, "Oh my God, am I going to die in Peru? What did I get myself into?" All kinds of thoughts ran through my head.

Opening my eyes, I looked up and saw millions of stars showering me with the most radiant light show I had ever seen, lighting up the darkness of the skies with luminescent sparkles. The stars felt so close, as if I could reach out my hand and just touch any star. After all, we were nearly 8,000 feet in the air on top of a mountain. I truly felt part of the universe, and, to the universe I would return one day, whenever that would be. I felt at peace.

As I lay there, open for any experience, I heard the shaman say, "When you are living your life so fully, with integrity and totality, feeling fulfilled, and THIS was your LAST moment, you'd be ready to die." (I wondered if Mark Twain knew anything about the shamans' way of approaching life and death. They sure had similar views). What a profound statement! What a profound notion! A lot to ponder, for sure.

Asking yourself what you want to feel in your last breath is a great question. If you're not feeling what you want to feel right now, it's time to pause. This could be your last breath. You just never know. I mean, don't we all want to feel blessed, loved, fulfilled, and grateful, with an overall sense of well-being and peace, happy with the life we've lived, feeling loved by our family and friends? I do, that's for sure.

I use this question with my clients. Many couples come to me and begin by telling me, "He did this, or she did that." "He said this, and she said that," and I inevitably ask them what their part is, and if this was his or her last breath, is this the way they want to go out? It stops them in their tracks and helps them put things in perspective.

When we feel in our hearts that we are actually making a difference by being alive, living in integrity, sharing who we are, and living from our soul's design, we feel in alignment with our "purpose". Our lives matter. We are making a difference in this world just by being who we were meant to be. Then, when "that" time comes, we can "go" knowing we made an impact. Wouldn't that just be the best?

That's why it's so important for us to live our lives as fully as possible now, to be who we want to be now, and not wait until "then," whenever "then" will be. Little did I know that this "conscious living and dying" awareness in Peru would plant a seed within me that would change my life forever.

For the past fifty or more years, as you have seen in your own life, time has a way of going faster the older we get, and if you keep everything you want to experience in the future, you're putting off your joy for another time. It's important to live a life that delights and surprises you now and brings you a deeper sense of well-being now.

That soothing, calming sense of well-being permeates from the inside out, letting you know, "Everything is okay... this human experience is a wondrous adventure, an exciting journey, a very special journey, even if it's challenging."

So, I ask you, are you living the life you love? IF this was your last breath, would you feel fulfilled, loved, grateful, and blessed, without regrets, and "ready to go" - because your life is so full? It's a good question to ask yourself. If you're not living the life you love now, ask yourself why not, and if not now, when?

After the West, we sojourned to the North, which is symbolized by the horse or dragon. It's the place to claim your mastery. The shamans always gather in a circle of 12, and in the crystal cave, where we had our ceremony, there are always 11 shamans sitting, with one open space for you to take your place in the circle with the wisdom you have to share. It's time to claim your mastery, to step into the circle of wisdom with what you know.

Finalizing the trip, we ventured to the East, represented by the eagle, who sees life from 5 miles high. The shamans always say that you are in the center of the Indian Medicine Wheel, and to look at your life from each direction gives you the perspectives you need to balance your life. There is no right or wrong, according to the shamans, only right or left.

In the East, we found ourselves at the Temple of Moon and were told to find a meditation spot on the terraced mountain. I found my spot and could feel the love from Mother Earth enter my body. Every cell of my being was filled with this love. I had so much love inside of me; it was oozing out, I could even "flick it off" my fingers. I felt the most peace I had ever felt in my entire life. Every fiber of my being was resonating with love.

I saw the shaman sitting at the bottom of the terrace and wondered to myself, "The shaman nurtures every single person, taking a dose of Ayahuasca for every dose a person takes, holding the space for them. Who nurtures the shaman?" Just as I was thinking this, I saw the shaman approach me and lay his head in my lap. I stroked his long hair, as a mother would a child and just held him, nurturing him, giving him my love.

I felt the power of love emanating from every pore of my being. As we got up, ready to return to our hotel, I felt as if I was floating off the ground, not even walking. I got onto the bus and sat in the back seat, and all of the shaman's apprentices came flocking to me, touching my legs and arms and nestling around me like kittens as I held them with my love. I had never experienced anything like that in my entire life.

I came back thinking my love could heal anything. I was wrong. I couldn't pry someone's heart open if they didn't want it opened. My husband felt threatened by my newfound empowerment of love, so I diminished it over time to "save" the relationship.

Flash forward to 2003. Diagnosed with breast cancer and facing divorce for the 3rd time after an almost 20-year marriage, I had to reinvent myself at 57 years old. I had to rediscover who I truly was. I had given up my empowered self, lost my identity, and was depressed.

No surprise, I was diagnosed with depression and given a prescription for Zoloft. Instead of relying on Zoloft for the depression. I took a 3-day course which changed my life. On the third day, I decided to invest $25,000 into their 4-year program that consisted of 5 outdoor survival courses. I found myself jumping off bridges on a bungee cord, repelling 2500' mountains, walking on coals, eating fire, laying on a bed of glass, and conquering my fears through might and love. Something in me was determined to rewire my brain and swore I would never have unhealthy relationships ever again. Thank God, to this day, I haven't.

I was becoming a full-time student of life, studying and receiving certifications in different coaching and training modalities, yearning to help others. I became my own best client and was blessed to coach others in what I had learned.

In 2005, one of my best friends, Susan, was dying of leukemia. She was 62 years old. She asked me to move in with her, her husband, and her 15-year-old son to help navigate the experience. Somehow, I knew I could guide them. All I can say is that "grace" stepped into me to help them navigate through it all with as much ease and grace as possible… and a lot of humor.

My instincts and comfort level surprised even me. I had to have done this type of work in a previous life. How else would I feel so comfortable with it all? Anyway, it was a mystery and a gift. What I learned in Peru many years ago kicked in big time.

On the 5th Monday, Susan's husband and I took her to her normal doctor's appointment at City of Hope. But this particular Monday was different. She told her doctor she had had enough. No more treatments.

The doctor told Susan how sorry she was and that she would do everything she could to make her as comfortable as possible. Susan even consoled the doctor back, saying, "It's not your fault. I know you did everything you could." We knew this was the beginning of the end, and I vowed to make it the most sacred healing experience ever.

On the way home, I suggested we have a gathering on Wednesday with her best girlfriends, she called her "sisters", so they could say goodbye and tell her how much they love her and her them.

She said, in her high-pitched New Jersey voice, as she slouched in the back seat like a little broken bird, "We can't have it on Wednesday. Cathy is a psychologist and has clients on Wednesday. Let's have it on Friday."

I said, "What if you die on Friday?" She exclaimed, "I'm going to die on Friday?" I said, "Well, I don't know, but if you did, wouldn't you be mad that you didn't have it on Wednesday? If people can drop what they are doing for a funeral, they sure as hell can drop what they're doing for a gathering." She said, okay.

It took me all of 20 minutes to gather the girls for Wednesday. One of them was even flying in from Kansas. We decked out Susan's dining room with all her favorite dishes and flowers, making the table look elegant and beautiful, just like she liked it. It became one of the most profound, meaningful, and healing gatherings for everyone!

I asked each woman to bring a small token, maybe a charm or a button or something of theirs, they could put in a small voile bag so she could take it with her, and to prepare something to say to her, letting her know how much they loved her and what an impact she made on their lives.

Each one came prepared and took turns facing her frail little body in her wheelchair. She was no longer able to walk, but believe me, she heard every word everybody said to her. Needless to say, we were all crying. It was one of the most touching and healing moments anybody had ever experienced.

After the brunch was over, we tucked her delicate, weakened body back into bed. That was the last time she was conscious. She died on Saturday.

During her last days, I continuously played soothing, calming music that transcended time and space. Sometimes, I would lay next to her and stroke her little bald head ever so gently, whispering encouraging words to her, wishing her well on her journey ahead, letting her know that she was loved and appreciated and that her life really mattered.

I'm not sure if you know this, but hearing is the last sense to go when someone is dying, so even though they may be unconscious, they can hear everything you are saying. Smell is the second to last sense to go. I sprayed one of her favorite scents, called, "Rain" into the air so she could smell the freshness and sweetness of life.

She indeed had a full life with her husband. They traveled around the world together, attended lectures, classical concerts, and book clubs, were very involved in the Jewish community, and, at 47 years old, she had the miracle baby she always wanted. She loved life!

On that Saturday morning, her husband had a meeting, and I was on watch. He suggested I keep the curtains closed and let her be quiet in the dark. It was a glorious day outside, with the sun shining and a bright blue sky. Something came to me, and I decided that if she was going to die today, she would go in the light and not the dark. I pressed that magical button, and the curtains opened like the Red Sea parting. Light began to pour into the room, and it was magnificent.

The best thing was that I could see her face. I noticed her grimacing, which meant she was uncomfortable or in pain, which I would not have seen had I kept the darkness alive. I realized that her organs shut down and were released in the bed. I would not have seen that either. I called the housekeeper to bring a bucket of warm, soapy water and some towels and told her we were going to clean her up. She was not going out in soiled clothes nor linens.

As I was cleaning her body, I felt like a midwife, just cleaning up a bigger baby. It was loving and sweet. I put on one of her favorite Prada shirts and scarves. I said to myself that she was going out with dignity, honor, and regard, and that's how her husband was going to see her when he returned.

I called her husband and the doctor, letting them know what was happening, and continued to play the music softly. The doctor arrived first and said he had never seen or felt anything like this before in all the 40 years he was a doctor, and it moved him to tears. We have a special bond to this day.

Her husband and I took turns sitting with her. He had left the room for a moment, and she let go of her last breath. It was such an honor and privilege to be present in that moment, to witness her life force leave her body, and THE most profound moment I had ever experienced.

When we are born, we are born with an inhale (spirit coming in) and when we die, we let go of our last breath with an exhale (spirit going out). It's as simple as that. Two breaths. What we do with all the breaths in between makes up the quality of our lives. We never know when that last breath will be.

So, how do you want your last breath to be? Do you want to feel loved and blessed? Grateful for your life? Fulfilled? Joyful? So full that you are ready to die? If so, start now. What are you waiting for? Take care of yourself and your body. Do something you love doing. Love the people you are with. Don't let time go by without telling someone you love that you love them. Why wait? Why wait to feel blessed?

Our human experience is a bumpy ride but also filled with unlimited opportunities to live as fully as we want. While we are here, we have the opportunity to cram in as many wondrous experiences into our lives as possible, reflecting the highest and greatest good, revealing the true majesty of the mysterious unknown, and enjoying ourselves.

Find the things/people in your life you are grateful for and appreciate every single part of your life now. You've got this! You can do it! You can live the life you love and love the life you live now!

About Shelley Whizin

Shelley Whizin, a seasoned joyful Transformational Life Coach, is revered for her profound understanding of the human-spiritual dynamic. Committed to uplifting women over 50, she inspires individuals to reconnect with their true values and infuses every moment with love and humor. Shelley empowers clients to transcend limitations and embrace well-being and fulfillment. Drawing from her own journey of resilience and reinvention following breast cancer and divorce at 57, her coaching is imbued with genuine care and empathy, illuminating paths to authenticity and joy. Shelley's coaching surpasses boundaries. With over three decades of experience, her impact extends beyond earthly realms, guiding clients through life's tender transitions with honor, grace, and wisdom to the very last breath and beyond.

Chapter Six

No One Ever Said Life Was Easy, But What a Wild Ride!

By: Denise Dalton, J.D

Each decade of life carries significance and can serve as a delineation in gauging one's progress. Introspectively, nearing the end of my fifties, I concur with those who have referred to this particular decade as the golden age of wisdom and experience, built upon a multitude of experiences from our past. For me, the fifties have marked a profound transformational period navigating the labyrinth of my own identity, increasingly shedding social expectations, and embracing my own true sense of self. I have persevered, adapted and bounced back from life's challenges and honed my resilience. Now, looking back on my own progress through my earlier decades of life, and particularly this latest one, I am increasingly looking forward to my sixties, armed with an even greater sense of freedom and liberation than I had entering my fifties.

As I approached my fifties, I had finally grown into a sense of personal power despite various obstacles and personal challenges I had encountered over the preceding thirty years of my adult life. I found my stride and an unyielding sense of self-confidence, knowledge and sound judgment, yet aware there was so much I still did not know but it was okay, and liberating. I was content with my career, physical strength and appearance, strong social connections and family, and feeling a sense of overall life satisfaction. Old insecurities would still arise, but they no longer controlled me. I was a kick ass attorney prosecuting complex financial fraud crimes in a highly skilled position at the Attorney General's Office. I loved my job and was on a trajectory to the top of my game. I anticipated my fifties to be a continuation of my life plan and even potentially a period of stable middle-age years. I was set, fully prepared for the future--or so I thought.

Then came my fifties, and what a wild and crazy yet wonderful ride it has been! As a younger woman, never in a million years could I have imagined that my fifties would be such an eventful decade. Writing this chapter has been a refreshing exercise of self-introspection as I now face down the big 6-0, I realize it may be that my fifties have been filled with more unexpected life experiences than I have experienced in any single decade thus far.

What a mix of emotions ranging from professional pride and success to the despair of sexual harassment and retaliation. From the confidence of physically athletic vitality and health to feelings of uncertainty and confusion of menopause and despondency. From the earlier joys of falling in love and motherhood, to the grief of losing loved ones. From the blissful oblivion of my own mortality to supporting my husband through unexpected major open-heart surgery and the pandemic.

My fifties include living abroad, learning a new language, culture, and way of life where I am developing a wide range of new friends, together with the life-enriching adventures and joys of traveling, including Summer and Fall seasons staying in different countries throughout Europe. No, my fifties have not been sedate or stable, and certainly not boring.

Reflecting on my life, I realize that my understanding of the importance of time began at an early age when I began competitive gymnastics. Competition taught me that time is relentless, always moving forward. I learned that the time between each competition was an opportunity for growth and improvement. This knowledge motivated me to perfect routines and challenge myself to learn increasingly difficult moves. If I did not seize each moment, I would waste precious time and remain stagnant. Time became my driving force toward success, my "True North." This concept of time became even more significant when setting and achieving future goals. Despite a career-ending injury as a young gymnast, I adapted by joining the gymnastics and diving teams, including dance squad and cheerleading in high school and college. Following my True North brought me great successes. I have also suffered consequences by losing focus and deviating from my True North. In essence, understanding the value of time and staying true to my goals has led me to achieve success – although it has not always been easy.

During my second year of college, I temporarily lost focus on my goals, but regained my path by working as a billing secretary while taking college courses during lunch breaks and evenings. I gradually made progress towards my degree and eventually became a legal secretary at a prestigious law firm. It was during this time that I met and married a young partner, blending our family together and immediately becoming a mother to four children. My husband's mother brought added challenges to our marriage. She carried insecurities from her son's previous divorce and held unrealistic expectations for her son's second marriage based on her insecurities and feigned religious beliefs. She was determined to "make me into a perfect supporting wife and mother" while putting my education on hold. Despite this, I had several wonderful years I will never regret. I continued to work but also used my training as a mediator and started a successful mediation practice, had two books published about blending families and teaching negotiation skills to children.

Towards the end of our marriage, I injured my knee protecting our daughter while snow skiing. The injury required surgery and a long recovery. Unfortunately, my mother-in-law insisted on staying with us to help, even though my own family lived nearby. Her unpredictable behavior added a new tension in our household. Little did I know that having my mother-in-law staying with us would result in a major turning point in my life.

While recovering from my surgery, my husband was emotionally drained and impulsively demanded a divorce while throwing his wedding ring at me. This shocking moment marked the beginning of a transformative journey for me. Though he later apologized and claimed he did not mean it, I knew our marriage could never fully recover. Determined to seek independence and pursue my dreams, I determined to complete my undergraduate degree and attend law school. Over the course of three years, I obtained my undergraduate degree while being a full-time student with a full-time job as a single parent of two young children. Although we tried to keep our marriage together for a few more years, it ended in divorce. Throughout this time, my focus remained on my children first and foremost. It was not an easy process, but I remained committed to my True North, prioritizing higher education, and working towards a better future.

I graduated from college with an impressive GPA but my performance on the law school admission test fell short of expectations. As a result, I faced rejections from schools I had applied to, except for being wait-listed at a prestigious West Coast institution. Rather than waiting another year, I decided to attend a lower-tiered law school in rural Ohio. Acquiring a legal education proved to be more challenging than anticipated. As a former legal secretary, I underestimated the demands of law school. Settling into a new state without a support system added to the difficulty. Despite these obstacles, we managed to navigate through together sharing memorable experiences. Balancing my studies with parenting was a daunting task. Finding time to study remained a constant struggle; after tucking the children in bed, I often studied early into the morning hours.

Weekends provided some respite as the children enjoyed activities at the public library while I focused on my studies. I also made sure to prioritize my children's well-being by enrolling them in personal training lessons and exploring outdoor activities together. Fortunately, my ex-husband remained a supportive figure, providing invaluable assistance while I pursued my education. During the first two years of law school, I achieved significant success and earned the opportunity to complete my final year as a visiting student at a law school in our hometown. Importantly, I developed a relationship with a man who became my fiancé and later my second husband. Together, we created a true 21st Century family, including the complexities of four children, each with different parents and visitation schedules during the time I was completing my third year of law school.

Upon graduating with a Juris Doctorate in Law, I faced the challenge of securing employment during an economic downturn. I was fortunate to join my ex-husband's private practice. Working alongside him provided me with valuable experience and opportunities to manage my own cases, represent clients in court, and defend a federal jury trial within my first year of practice. My passion for criminal law led me to pursue a position as a public defender, where I gained extensive courtroom experience overseeing various criminal cases. This experience paved the way for a more specialized role in the Attorney General's Office, prosecuting complex financial crimes and capital punishment cases. Although initially intimidating, I dedicated extra hours to research and sought guidance from supervisors and mentors. Through these efforts, I developed confidence and a solid foundation in my position and career.

Entering my fifties, I was the sole female prosecutor in the financial crimes division of the Attorney General's Office. I excelled in taking cases to trial, working closely with law enforcement and expert witnesses. Building rapport with victims and witnesses became a rewarding aspect of my work. With a flawless trial conviction record, I felt accomplished and secure in my position. As I approached the milestone fifty, I knew without a doubt I had found my true calling and this was it!

Over the years I cultivated numerous friendships with colleagues, including a close friend and mentor, who held the top non-elected position in the office. Despite our significant age gap, we formed a good friendship, and I appreciated his guidance. Both of us single at the time, socialized outside of work, attending social and work events together. Our relationship was strictly platonic. Then, during a Christmas holiday, my friend and I went out for a festive dinner. To my surprise, when he dropped me off that evening, he made an unwelcome advance by attempting to kiss me. I immediately made it clear that I did not reciprocate his romantic interest. Unfortunately, this incident had serious repercussions.

Upon returning to the office after the holidays, I discovered that a large rug I loaned to him for his office had been removed from his office and carelessly thrown in the doorway of my own office. Additionally, shared files, books and Christmas gifts had been haphazardly discarded on top of the rug. My entire team and staff were aware that something had transpired between us. The situation only worsened from there. My former friend began to ignore me in the hallways and started spreading malicious rumors about my abilities as an attorney to colleagues, who held him in high regard. Despite their subordination to him, they were influenced by his disparaging comments. His behavior in our weekly case review meetings became increasingly hostile. He would undermine my contributions by rolling his eyes, making derogatory remarks, or even physically turning away from me. These actions were far from subtle and quickly spiraled out of control. To make matters worse, he abruptly withdrew from our planned joint trial, leaving me with minimal time to prepare for the aspects of the case he would have handled. Nevertheless, I persevered and successfully tried the eight-week fraud case on my own, securing a conviction. Shortly thereafter, I noticed a significant shift in the assignments I received. The complex financial fraud cases that I had previously been entrusted with were no longer assigned to me. I was treated as an outsider and actively avoided by my colleagues. It was a horrific experience that caused my once-promising career to plummet.

What made it even more difficult was my reluctance to stand up for myself due to my former friend's high-ranking position. I feared the consequences of speaking out and losing my job. Moreover,

58

I grappled with the fact that I willingly fostered a friendship with this individual for years and worried that I would somehow be held responsible for the aftermath. My self-assurance and pride suffered a significant blow. Despite the immense difficulty I faced, I knew I had the resilience to prove to everyone that I would not be broken. Internally, however, I was slowly crumbling. It was time for a reassessment.

During this tumultuous period, I confided in my second husband, from whom I had been divorced twelve years earlier, but it was widely known we maintained an on-and-off relationship. To my astonishment, he revealed his intention to run for the position of Attorney General against my boss. Unfortunately, his timing could not have been worse for me. I attempted to dissuade him from pursuing his campaign, but he remained determined. As a member of the opposing political party, his chances of winning a statewide election were slim. Nonetheless, he forged ahead.

I chose to remain at the Attorney General's Office for almost a year. However, it had become increasingly unbearable. The fact that my second husband was running a political campaign against my boss only heightened the tension. He had asked me to assist him with the campaign, and while I considered the potential opportunities it could bring, I also recognized that there might be other paths ahead for me to explore. I conducted an honest assessment of my life, and it was clear that I had no control over my current work situation but did possess control over my own actions and decisions. I realized I had reached my breaking point.

Now in my mid-fifties, it was time to realign myself with my True North. I made the difficult decision to resign, expressing gratitude in my resignation letter to those who had supported me along the way. However, I intentionally omitted any mention of the man who had harassed and retaliated against me, as a subtle way of shedding light on the mistreatment I had endured. It was a challenging decision, but it taught me a valuable lesson: never again will I relinquish my power or allow my voice to be silenced. I have emerged from this experience with a renewed sense of self-confidence and a steadfast commitment to advocating for myself and others, standing up against any form of harassment or mistreatment.

After resigning, my second husband and I opted to rekindle our relationship and exchange vows once more. With the culmination of my resignation and his political campaign, we began devoting more time to our cozy home in Mexico, engaging in remote legal work. As we settled into our newfound routine, I embarked on an exhilarating endeavor to reimagine and renovate our house. To my astonishment, I renewed my ardor for this form of artistic pursuit. While my husband was comfortable speaking Spanish, I undertook the task of learning the language and adapting to the different lifestyle in our adopted village. Our shared aspiration to explore uncharted territories and establish roots overseas has perpetually propelled us forward.

Despite my spouse embracing retirement, I harbored no intentions of retiring just yet. We resolved to take a brief hiatus, allowing ourselves to fully immerse in our aspirations and seize the moment, particularly amidst the unprecedented challenges of the pandemic. Our quest for thrill and novelty led us down unforeseen avenues, presenting a mélange of unforeseen trials and serendipitous blessings. During our sojourn in Mexico, I was in a life-altering auto-accident. A speeding truck collided with the driver's side of my vehicle resulting in my sustaining severe concussions and narrowly avoided paralysis, in addition to an assortment of other wounds. As I embarked on the arduous path to recovery, my partner confronted his own health ordeal from rupturing of two heart valves. In a race against time, I hastily drove him two hours inland to a hospital, where it took five days to stabilize him. Once he received medical clearance, we flew home to the United States, and he underwent intricate open-heart surgery with an extended convalescence in the hospital. This traumatic episode had a profound impact on both of us, yet it also fortified our conviction that it was not our destiny to die that year. We both recovered and rode out the pandemic in our secluded idyllic Mexican fishing village on the beach where we forged cherished memories and found respite during the global crisis. Once travel restrictions were lessened, we eagerly resumed our peripatetic travels. Our intrepid spirits persistently propel us forward as we embrace the still unknown of wonders and rich diversity that the world has to offer.

As I approach the end of my fifties, I eagerly anticipate my next career venture with the freedom to explore opportunities worldwide, without being confined by location. The multitude of choices can be overwhelming, but having options is always positive. Although I no longer look or feel like I did in my thirties, I am confident in my ability to adapt and overcome any challenges that come my way. I firmly believe that I can achieve any goal I set for myself, guided by my unwavering determination. There are moments when I take pride in the wrinkles and smile lines on my face, as they are a testament to the experiences I have lived through. There are also times, however, when I catch a glimpse of my mother's reflection in the mirror and feel a sense of horror. In such instances, I am open to utilizing treatments like botox and fillers to address any concerns. The concept of "aging gracefully" is so very subjective, and every woman has the freedom to decide her own path. We each have our own unique ways of navigating the challenges of Mother Nature, who can be a bitch at times.

Being active has always been a significant part of my life. As I find myself closer to sixty than fifty, there are moments I feel as energetic as a twenty-year-old, while at other times, not so much. Nevertheless, over the past five and a half decades, I have found joy in the same activities and more. (Currently, I am writing this chapter from my hometown in the mountains, surrounded by falling snow, springtime skiing is calling to me.) It is more crucial than ever to prioritize regular exercise and maintain a healthy diet, as I intend to continue being active and participating in the sports and activities I love for as long as possible. I learned the hard way that once muscle mass is lost, rebuilding it becomes a significant challenge. I am not particularly fond of the way my body has changed or the saggy skin that has appeared, but I am actively making the necessary changes I can and accepting those that are beyond my control.

If I had the opportunity to travel back in time and enlighten my thirty-five-year-old self about the experiences of menopause (something I had no knowledge of at the time), I would offer her the following advice: Menopause is not for the faint-hearted. The symptoms are a natural part of the process, but changes will occur. Do not feel embarrassed or allow anyone to shame you for what you are experiencing. Emotional and physical changes will begin to manifest in your late forties. It may not always make sense, and others may not be understanding of the challenges you are experiencing. Brain fog and anxiety are real and should not be dismissed. You are not losing your mind or becoming paranoid, even though it may feel that way. Stay strong, stand your ground, and always advocate for yourself. Do not let challenges bring you down. You will have unexpected emotions and mood swings. Hot flashes and night sweats are real and can persist for years. Seek treatment for the migraines you are about to experience, get a doctor who will take the time to understand your needs. Keep spare clothing in your office and car, as you may experience unexpected menstrual gushes. Your hair, eyelashes, and eyebrows will thin. Remember that you are not alone on this journey. Do not allow your male colleagues to dismiss your opinions or position by making derogatory remarks about "that time of the month" or menopause. Put an end to that immediately! Learn from your friends, spouse and chosen family, as they are invaluable sources of support, and you need each other. Never forget your strength, and always be proud of who you are.

Lastly, I must express my deepest gratitude for the incredible and supportive family of choice I have built throughout my life. These relationships are founded on deep friendships, love, and unwavering support among a core group of women, many of whom I met in college and others who have come into my life over the years. These strong, independent, and successful women love and trust each other unconditionally. While we may have different perspectives and occasional intense disagreements, we never lose sight of the unwavering love we share. Together, we navigate the various stages of this unpredictable, remarkable, and sometimes challenging journey called life. We share both the pain and the joy life brings. Some of us have traveled, moved away, or even live in different countries, but we always maintain our connections and hold one another in our hearts. We embrace playfulness, adventure, and find ways to spend time together whenever possible. I am grateful for my family of choice, as they are my role models, heroes, and my angels. We forge ahead together into the unknown, facing whatever challenges come our way with strength and determination. I cherish every moment spent with these incredible women. I love you all deeply and will forever be grateful for the bond we share. Together, we will conquer the world and create a legacy that will inspire generations to come.

Here's to all of us living an unapologetically audacious and fabulous life!

About Denise Dalton, J.D:

Denise Dalton, J.D., is a former prosecutor of financial crimes and received her undergraduate degree in Sociology. When they are not traveling, she and her husband are currently enjoying their lives together in a small Mexican fishing village overlooking the Pacific Ocean. They are eagerly anticipating more of life's never-ending adventures and are preparing for their next travel experiences abroad.

Chapter Seven
Multi Faceted Diamond
by Aryana Congdon

I was so looking forward to turning 50, it sure had an energy that I soooo didn't feel at 40, a new time and clearer journey and oh so many possibilities. It felt like a clean slate, magical in a way and I could feel my soul's light. It was a gift yet to be revealed and I had excitement.

Not long into my 50's I was side swiped! Something from my outside environment entered my space. The words the perpetrator used was "Welcome to your day of Devastation!"

Wow didn't see that coming. So began a different journey through "my" 50's with all its 5's as 5 represents change in numerology.

In short, the charges were kidnap and rape. It went through the courts with the main case being heard nearly 2 years later. As you can image there was times of dark and times of light, not sleeping, not wanting or being able to get out of bed, PTSD, anxiety, starvation and emotional eating, hair falling out, not being able to go out in public in the beginning because I would end up rocking in tears on the floor of the supermarket struggling to breathe. Not able to read anything, my eyes could not see the words mostly and if they did, I could not retain the previous word (I am now reading and comprehending words in my own way) while finishing raising my son.

He had to appear as a witness and have 3 days in court and after the Guilty verdict the very next day was his 18th birthday.

We had an amazing party at the house with my beautiful people around us and his around him. We had treasure hunts, games, food and laughter. A young man from our antenatal group came up to me and was telling me all the things he had been up to. I asked him how come I didn't know this? After a pause he replied, "You were busy." I looked into his eyes of full love and compassion and told him I will never be too busy for his adventures again. From that moment I felt PRESENCE. I felt a shift and that I could again be in life with my friends and family and be in their life's adventures. Their joy was my joy while finding mine again for me.

Old family sayings came back to me.

From my son's 18th birthday, my first saying became, "Celebrate everything, the good, bad and the ugly!" I have to say I found this to be quite light and it sometimes caused me to laugh, partly because what else was there to do and partly because it can't get any worse lol.

Sometimes this caused "silly dancing" too which really was doing a Taylor Swift and shaking it off. One of my father's sayings was, "If you have lost your humour, you have lost everything" ... so very true and I do give thanks 'cos I find it does always come back and I found "out of bad there is always good," one of my mother's sayings. So very true, traversing through Chaos, to get to peace. Each part of my journey that was Chaos could not be going around it or over it, it had to be me going through it. A walk in the shadows.

As a child I was scared of the dark. I would feel and see things that some people wouldn't, terrified and stricken at times and your adults saying, there is nothing there, it's alright, go back to sleep.

On the internet, Survivors of rape hold a board up in front of them with most of their face hidden, with words the perpetrator said to them that they will never forget from that experience. The words he told me were, "YOU WILL NEVER GET OVER THIS IF YOU DON'T LOSE THE FEAR." Hmmmm what to do with that one, weird info to me, he could do all he did and leave me with the key to get through?

So, I realized this journey is into the dark and shadow, into Fear and is as long as a piece of string (which a beloved sister said and which annoyed me at times to hear it again and again because of the truth of it).

When seeing in front of me I saw the string with no end in sight at that time and when I looked behind me there was nothing there, it was dissolved and did not exist, a sign I was moving through it.

So being in this awareness of a walk into the shadows and to befriend the dark, I came across an Oracle card with a Shadow Queen. You could call on her and she would walk with you into the dark while holding space, she never spoke as this was my discovery. I would call her in a meditation or dream space because I had answers to seek. She always turned up and greeted me with a smile and I would take her arm. Over the years I did not call on her as much, as I could walk in myself, in confidence and knowing that the unknown will present itself as a spark of light, and so my answers were now known. My journey with fear, dark, shadows, unknown and then known. The tool that got me through was befriending the fear by becoming a frenemy to a friend.

The perpetrator and the Chaos that he had bought into my world, was an outside of me thing. That took me inside to all my bodies, physically, mentally, emotionally, and spiritually. I just could not understand the Unkindness (as I labelled it). I found that I was never going to understand something I am not, so this knowledge brought me out of that looping that was programming my head.

Then there was forgiveness. I didn't innerstand this either, it did not make sense to me, there was actually nothing to forgive. It had happened and was it something I had created? Or meant to have happened? Yes. So, to change it I would say to myself, thank you for giving me this experience to move on from what was not serving me. I saw through the court his journey and his looping, that was his and his was not mine.

Now when fear comes in to present itself, I talk to the energy and fear gives me all the information I need to let go and move it on. An insightful friend indeed.

What I have found with my 50's journey that I was gifted with, is that there's so many layers and expansiveness. What I believed then I do not now believe as you peel off the layers to another innerstanding, you keep going deeper and deeper much to your soul's delight and therefore change is always happening. You surf the wave of change to the shore and the next wave comes in for another change of your multifaceted self.

Innerstanding and peeling back the layers as they are now known to you then becomes your wisdom. When you resist the change, you become static and sometimes stuck in your stuff/shit. S H I T (look closer at this word: expand it out).   S H I F T.... shit doesn't happen yet shifts do.

One of the shifts I had to make through this experience was with a color. I call myself a "color slut", lol, 'cos I just adore color, my grandmothers and mother too loved color and were always admiring the colors of nature herself, of fabrics and furnishings. There was no prejudice to color, all were loved and seen and accepted while each one of them had their favorite hues. I have never had a favorite and love mixing it up hence the self title of color slut. My pregnancy color was yellow, I wore a lot of it then and now I'm so happy.

With what I had survived I noticed that orange was becoming unfavorable and triggered me. I had a prejudice with orange! Besides the emotional triggers it caused was the sadness of this insight. I worked out that on that day he had worn orange, that I remembered, or maybe it was the color that triggered these meltdowns, as I called them. I also began noticing that my favorite dress was orange! Wow how opposite. I began to see that when orange was in front triggering me, the orange I was wearing was healing me, making me aware of how I felt about orange. This showed me that orange was nothing to do with this, it was neutral with no prejudice. I remembered with all of me that orange was love and gorgeousness and everywhere in mother nature. It was like mother nature was with me too. By seeing the colors she represented and the flowers beside each other I could understand that everything goes with everything. I was not alone, mother nature was with me too, like the beautiful beloved souls and spirit walking with me.

Being the color of the sacral chakra and a place where emotions can be stored, orange took me on a rocky road to begin with, discovering emotions that turned to feeling the feelings. This adds a space for you to become the observer and see in an expansive vision, the truth of it. This was one of the teachings from trees for me.

I could then go to the wardrobe in a neutral space and allow my inner me or my body to choose today's colored outfit. When it was orange, I would put it on and feel embraced like a big hug, then magic would happen from the universe. When I went out and came across someone wearing orange in front of me, I would feel the trigger inside me much lessened until it was not there anymore. I focused on the orange I was wearing, the feeling of the hug and embrace and I could feel both oranges were the same thing, one outside me and one on and inside me. From being triggered to feeling joy of color again and then to conscious dressing, looking in the mirror, some kind of self love was growing and also my hair which then led to my personal style coming back. I was coming back from the inside out! Woo Hoo.

Underneath the clothes was another layer to the journey... my body. Funny how we blame ourselves to any percent of big or small. That can lead to a variety of addictions as we go through our journey. Within a week of the attack, I was in the dreamtime in a more conscious state, when my breasts came to me and in a very clear voice said, "Don't blame us! He enjoyed us." What? I thought. Yup I had heard right. I told them that I did not remember that. "That's why we are telling you. You weren't always in your body, so your memory is different to ours," they said. Well, I had to sit with that one for a moment. Then I called to my vagina, "How are you after all that?"

Quickly she came back to me, "Like you, I took a bit of a bashing! But I'm ok, how are you?" she said. Omg I'm talking to my vagina and breasts I'm thinking. Yes, we both took a bit of a bashing I confirmed. From there we had a chat about my emotions which my body parts were completely neutral about. My body parts saying don't blame us, was astounding and I have to say I realized long after that I wanted to blame some part of me, the body me. I don't remember at this time blaming the perpetrator, I guess I labelled him unkind because I remember everyone I knew and my experiences had mostly been kind, so I labelled him unkind. I realize I was just putting the blame on me and trying to place it on my body somewhere. My vagina invited me into her whenever I needed to talk or just to be held in a womb like mother nature or in a quiet space of No-Thingness, to BE. When I went into her in meditation, she became this very luscious red, soft as a couch, so delicious, vibrant and nurturing, the color of passion for me. So, I renamed her my 'passion pit'. When I feel like visiting from that day to this, I feel so loved and supported. She would just BE with ME, (My Energy). I would always ask her what she needed if anything - sometimes she would answer that she required vitamins or minerals or a kind loving thought towards her as I walked through my day. Mostly she would say just love me. From there we talk of anything I might like to do, to create or to manifest. That's what a passion pit does, create, from the cauldron or chalice of your base chakra. She teaches me many things and our conversations are vast topics since we have connected more.

After the first initial conversation I decided to get a wax. It felt very private to me and for us. One evening, when with a bunch of friends, I can only describe as luscious goddesses of a table filled with nectars... the conversation came up about those that wax. They were all in favor of being natural and could not understand waxing and Brazilian etc. The conversation went around the table to say who has 'what hairstyle down there?' I told them I waxed it off, I was the only one in the room who had. They all stared at me until my curious friend asked why. So, I took a breath and said, "Well, since the rape I just need to see my vagina so I can see that she's alright."

I felt stupid saying it, the room paused. Then they all spoke at once, they understood why I had, and I could feel them in themselves considering their vaginas.

This brought about a few things, a beautiful goddess connection and a deeper sharing of their heart truths and sometimes pain and always in all ways strength. I saw bravery again; I saw that when you share in a loving space that all is accepted and acknowledged and it's ok to ask why.

On one of my visits to my passion pit I was explaining how tired bleeding made me feel as my period had always been 7 days, heavy and starting at 13. I asked her if she would mind stopping them and if she did that the lovely uterus would remain with me til the earthly body was no more, and that she would remain healthy and let me know of any needs. She said she would stop it and was happy to comply. She had to go for a photoshoot a few years after that and I asked to see the scan. There she was, regal, with the fallopian tubes all tucked in and all was peace filled. I was in deep gratitude and felt her presence. The medical staff labelled it post menopause.

Before the scan, years before, another talk around my women friends was menopause. I so was not on this page with all I had going on, however I listened to them. They were really querying this as it could happen at any stage, and they were looking for more fitting and expansive information. I could feel my ancestors at this time and what they had been through. Theirs was labelled "Hysteria" so connecting with the doctors' long list of possible ailments along with my feminine ancestors, I really felt this Man-made list. Well, that was it! No way was I going through that! So, I changed the name and reclaimed my power, "A PAUSE IN MEN!", that was what I was traveling through, throwing out the patriarchal bs. While taking a pause in men also, I remained on my "inside" journey. (Just so you know I'm through my "pause in men" now.) For me, it's been about the stress in the body through the journey, the cortisol etc which I am still discovering. So really, I just really chose to stick to talking to my body….. a never-ending voyage.

Growing up my mother and her friends had a "Spinning Group", it did start out at that, and they did keep doing their creative projects, fine sherry and food and cups of tea. They would share their inner truths sometimes to each other, as some were still of the old ancestral school of privacy. Our mother would share information with us of the goddess nature, so that things were not hidden or secret as far as she was able to within her limits. And so we grew up as younger women from this sharing circle.

When, through the beginning of this journey my sister arrived from another city, we did the usual let's go to a café thing. As we walked along the path there were a flock of people heading towards us, as they got closer, they all Smiled! to me…my sister said, 'Did you see that?' Oh yes, it was spirit, it felt like a celebration of maybe getting through the last few days, I don't know, just that I remembered the power of a smile. As a teenager I was often told that I smiled too much. It was just showing my appreciation of the moment. Well. this experience brought back the smile, the power of it and how people you walk pass or come in contact with treasure, a SMILE.

After that, friends found out what had happened to me. They came to me in their own space and time. I told them to tell their children, because I didn't see or feel the need to hide this. I think it was that whatever happens to them in life they would be supported, in their re-remembering. One by one my friends came to me, and we shared time … a great gift. They would bring the most heartfelt gifts, it still astounds me at this KINDNESS, (as I had to re-remember and accept kindness again while making peace and acceptance of unkindness). Some gifts were made by hand, one in particular was a reworked petticoat, embroidered with felt and flowers for my lady garden, angels to watch my back, a sun where my butt hole is lol. The gifts surprised me because I watched my friends from a witness/observer place. It was not just what they did or bought, it was their compassion and kindness, their creative artistry of themselves and their beautiful hearts. During these shared times their stories began to come out of their buried trauma histories of which I had no idea, a lot of these from some age in childhood. I think firstly that there were so many of them, it was like who hasn't had a perpetrator! This just rendered me speechless. And yet love expanded, compassion and a connection of souls sharing. This all came out before the time this was to go to court.

I remember the police taking me into the station afterwards and I was trying to cry softly. I was getting annoyed with this and so I asked myself why, the answer came back in words and pictures, because somewhere all over the world right now this is happening to men, children, and women, it hasn't stopped! I don't know why I felt this.

There were 2 things that happened from this.

The first is that just before the trial I rang everyone who had shared with me their stories. I invited them to walk with me through the trial. (As NONE of their perpetrators got reported let alone arrested or held accountable). To pretend, if they could not feel that, to imagine they were taking their perpetrator to court along with mine that day. That we will all walk together and receive the healing we needed at that time. At court we were given a room to wait in until I was called to the stand. My beautiful friends and family set up that room with magazines, board games, food, coffee, and tea in flasks etc... They made it ours. It was a very special sacred sharing space for us all, it flowed in love's energy and respect for all. At the end of the hearing when we got the GUILTY plea, I remember some dropping to the floor crying. Those who walked with me as a collective all said they felt healing from taking their perpetrator to court. What an amazing feeling of being all together and feeling our strength, I really still can't put this in words but I do know that love grew that day.

The second event was me taking myself off to my adopted mama. This was before trial. I went because I had to have a change of scenery and of course mama's food and nurturing was a drawcard too lol. I had so many emotions in me that were not shifting and my soul called me up north. In the long hours at mama's healing room I sat, wanting to write something, then my soul asked what is it you want. I told her my intention, picked up the pen and flowing from me came the intention/prayer.

I posted this on social media, and within 2 days a friend rang me and told me that the prayer had reached South India, a place where outcast women and dogs lived! They all lived together, and each day would wander the streets and pick up those who had been thrown out of their homes, animals now unwanted, women because of course it was often their fault in that culture? My friend told me that he had a message from this group in India. He had no idea how they got their intention/prayer so was a bit stumped himself to be contacted and yet handed on the message. "We could not believe that a sister so far away in the southern hemisphere understands us and gets it. Tell her we will be saying her prayer together at our morning prayer time." Wow.

I cried and could not believe it really, and yet it is true, I felt those sister's and the furry 4-legged beings. I felt a lot at that moment. I saw and witnessed connection, love, the power of intention, the magic we carry, the bigness of an intention and its ripple. I saw and felt we are never alone; we are always supported. That part in me is that part in you. Community, respect, gratitude....

So, 50 and fabulous? It's been a trip, it's been amazing. To have journeyed, to have turned all of it into knowledge, to share whole heartedly with compassion and kindness with beautiful souls and they with me, to pay it forward and to see and witness magic, to travel into the spaces within and to bring to light the wisdom. To keep moving forward and bring out gifts of my soul and expansion of that creatrix and to dance my dance of ME, (My Energy), in beauty and grace and remain true to all that I AM inside and weave my earth walk, in Joy. To be in the new freedom of my uniqueness and to rock my rhythm while still discovering the alchemy of living.

A PRAYER FOR HUMANITY

Preparation: Take 3 deep breaths to feel the connection to the prayer. When you are ready, say the intention/prayer out loud. This can also be done as a meditation.

I align with my higher self and soul

I am connected in the universal oneness of being

I am connected with the clear Intention of myself and others exponentially

I am connected to mother earth's core in peace and harmony

I am connected with all living things

TAKE 3 DEEP BREATHS

I call on the God force energy and that of St Germain's Violet flame

I ask for every person and living thing who have suffered at the hands of another, past and present,

That their hearts be open to receive the enlightenment and healing,

Through all times, dimensions and planes and on all levels, energies and bodies…

Place them in the memory of forgiveness of one's self,

Place them in the memory of understanding and higher learning,

Place them in their truth and the acceptance of their truth,

Place them in the knowledge to see the gift of rebirth and the opportunity of their wholeness healed,

Place them in their memory of strength, courage, beauty and grace, to continue to move forward into the light.

With Gratitude we thank you for the connection and alignment each soul seeks in their I AM PRESENCE.   SO BE IT

About Aryana Congdon

A student of life and life's journey and the people you meet on the way. A degree in art, published poet. I love the creative energy and seeing how that comes out of me and the continuous exploration of this. To celebrate everything, the good, the bad and the ugly. I also hold space for others, to empower and shine and bloom into their expansiveness through readings, healings and meditations etc. My website is www.aryana.co.nz

Chapter Eight

On Letting Go & Claiming Your Own Fabulous

by Dinny Lansdowne

Notes on embracing the power of choice, connecting to your true self, and activating your unique success frequency to create with ease, grace, and a wee bit of grit.

"It works if you work it, so work it, you're worth it" - overheard in NYC, back in the day. I was a Canadian fashion designer living on the Upper East Side in a five-story walk-up. The location was amazing, the apartment itself less than glam (facing the Bloomie's loading dock), and the last time I walked by, it had been torn down, just a lot with nine-foot weeds awaiting a post-pandemic reinvention. Everything changes, and my "what works" sure has too. My "what works if you work it" - at the time was to run flat out and keep on running. Fueled by meditation, adrenaline, and the buzz of the city, seeking creative expression in a business I had come to realize wasn't about that at all... I was pioneering a designer, eco-friendly, sweatshop-free fashion line that embraced body positivity and diversity.

Other than shifting into my intuitive, creative flow state for inspiration and guidance for design, marketing or strategy, I was in "get 'er done" mode, making so many connections and decisions it was a bit of a blur.

Downtime didn't exist. We were selling wholesale to 100s of stores as well as manufacturing and retailing back in Vancouver. I was wearing high heels and so many hats it's amazing I didn't topple over - designing collections, stores, photoshoots, manufacturing, trade shows, conscious messaging, marketing, PR, hiring, managing reps and retail staff, and on and on... staying ahead of the curve.

Looking back at my younger self, I bet I would have said "Of course, I'm choosing how to be and what to do!" Now, I have a wider lens and a long distance perspective. I see both the amazing results and successes and how narrow my focus was and what a high cost I paid. I was high energy, full on, even while pushing through some major health challenges.

I didn't aspire to be a designer while I was growing up. Backpacking around Asia after university sparked my interest. In Bangkok, I encountered the richest of linens, silks, and jacquard patterns in endless rainbows of colors. I discovered I could make a sketch and have a tailor transform it into a gorgeous garment that fit like a glove. I was hooked. It was a turning point and felt like the perfect way to combine creative expression and business. I didn't know what I didn't know (which was almost everything) and went headlong into designing with an agenda to create positive change in an industry that thrives on toxicity. I can feel the adrenaline rush even as I write this. Ick.

Long story short, I was so focused on being a change agent and leading-edge designer while trying to make my personal relationships work, that when I finally hit the wall, it was brutal. Thanks to a physical reality check I couldn't think my way out of - or overcome at high speed - I found myself face to face with me, myself, and I... and radical choice. The truth was not only the awesome press version everyone else saw. I had a gorgeous store, shipped to 100s of stores across Canada and the US, lots of press and TV, agents, awesome manufacturers, my home team in Vancouver, and... was always on the financial edge trying to collect, keep up and grow fast. With awesome support from my family, closest friends, staff and team, I made it through a couple of seasons I can barely remember, sometimes too weak to even walk. Something had to change. I had to decide if and how I was going to live.

I closed my business with a notice to our wholesale agents and stores, an award-winning "Clean Sweep Sale" window display, and made sure all my staff was placed. Fast flow as usual. Afterward, I felt like I had lost everything all at once, in all ways. My health, relationships with my significant other and step kids, my business, my store, my home, a connection with my industry colleagues.

 Luckily, before my hard stop, my press coverage had created demand for consulting, and I was directing brand, PR and business strategy for creative entrepreneurs on the side. This wasn't the first time I had lost it all…and I knew that failure opened doors, but at the time it was exhausting, dreadful, soul-crushing and I was physically frail. I rejected all "chronic" labels and as those have never matched my personal story or energy.

It was time to recalibrate, rethink, refuel and feel into what I might want next. Something we also do as we enter into our 50s and beyond.

Putting my health first and letting go of the garment industry was a big dramatic change, a wake-up call, and not the last one. I wish I could say I only had to learn to pay attention to my health once. It's been a life-long learning experience. Over the years, I've finally learned to pay attention to all areas of my life and notice what's working and what's signaling change. I've become attuned to tiny clues and now I pay attention.

The call to change may start as a faint whisper, but with time and awareness, it becomes undeniable. Whether it is a call to say, "No to!" or a shift forward to "Go To!", attuning to a call presents a fabulous opportunity - a moment for pausing and choosing what's next.

Following that call is a common theme among my clients. As CEOs, founders, transformational leaders, and creative change-makers, tuning into what is meant to be born is essential to their soul-path work, as it is for me. When you start noticing that decisions are driven by other people's demands, reactions, necessities, urgency, and deadlines… it may be a call. Or when you just aren't feeling great… what's going on? When your instinct is to shy away, what are you being told? When everything is going great, what else might be even more fabulous?

Even in the midst of organized chaos, I was always listening and watching for what might be next. I love connecting to a higher frequency and intuiting or downloading what's next. The call might be to walk away or perhaps to change something that's not working. It could be for an inspiring new direction. That's what launched my first major collection.

What I've learned, and practice consistently, is to be curious and always be noticing what is, what works, and what requires recalibration. Being interested sure beats the alternative. And pays off.

Sometimes it's the contrast between where I am, how I'm being and what I desire, that alerts me to the call. Maybe it's a negative thought. Or maybe I go straight to feeling something is off.

In these times, a quick inner check works. Or taking the time to shift and ground, letting the contrast dissolve into a oneness with all. To bask in the light and feel the spaciousness and possibilities just waiting to be called upon and activated.

In addition to blocking sacred space for meditating, creating, downloading or dreaming, I find spaciousness in the tiniest corners, in the few alone-in-the-midst-of-chaos moments, sitting with a coffee and a notebook in a crowded coffee shop, or while waiting at an announcement-blasting airport gate.

Another practice I count on is future casting. Getting balanced, calling in the light, grounding in gratitude, feeling into my success frequency (aka. Future Fabulosity!) and imagining what's next. This makes creating feel timeless and easier, no matter what is going on around.

Over the years, it's become a habit to notice and do my best to make a choice that works better. It's a way to avoid defaulting into old patterns that no longer work. It's automatic for me to get grounded and shift my state into my spacious, power place. (Actually, that's saved me from suffering many times.) And I absolutely count on the gift of asking for inspiration, what I must know, what my most effortless, strategic next path might be.

Before it sounds like everything is always one flowy, shiny experience, let me clarify: It's not as if it's all one way or the other, good or bad, or whatever label. I've certainly experienced being in a high vibe place and challenged at the same time. On the one hand my health, relationship, or location time may be challenged and yet I'm fast flowing on a project, jamming with clients or feeling totally inspired.

This has been true during many new ventures like art directing, producing, and styling on-location photoshoots, producing huge, multi-day entrepreneur education events, growing an agency engineering conscious business transformations, learning more healing modalities, traveling, and moving to sunny places.

I've used energy medicine and my favorite modalities to overcome pain and carry on, as well as heal. It took yet another major health crisis before I really recalibrated. It was time to truly tune into what might be even more fabulous for me on all levels. Once again, a crisis was the catalyst, but this time I decided to keep my branding and marketing company - Inspired Source Media Inc. - running.

I was unwilling to "lose it all" again, to let down and let go of my team, my clients, my revenue, and the momentum for positive impact. I paused to restructure, cutting down my time by over 90%.

Another fabulous result was my net income went way up and my team stepped up too. All of me was demanding and calling for more space, for more of a dynamic balance. And I had it for a while.

Was the choice to pause, to listen (especially when I didn't like what I was hearing) easy? No! Sometimes, it seemed that changing would cause me to lose everything, or at least a lot. This happened quite recently when I was experiencing spinal nerve pain that literally stopped me in my tracks. When life is flowing along beautifully, there always seem to be lots of awesome excuses for not pausing or stopping to redesign.

You probably have some reasons too. Both momentum and underlying fear are great excuses for saying I can't. Can't stop. Can't pause. Can't say no. Can't go. Can't leave. Can't stay. Can't change yet. Can't can't can't. Can't is closely related to "I have to do this"… and this and this too.

On the other hand, I have clients who are choosing to change so rapidly that are completely focused on "I can" and strategic action. Sometimes they don't pause, look back, nor give themselves enough credit. It's super common when you're always going for the next. Been there a few times.

Another time it's difficult to fully commit to change is in a situation that's mostly fabulous, but perhaps not working in some way. It takes grace, guts, grit and a huge dose of gratitude for what is, to shift from an "almost ok", "i can handle it" version of what works, to what works even better.

I'm still not brilliant at actively pursuing what I deeply desire when it conflicts with other areas of my life. Pretty sure I'm not alone in that. When I'm ok with what I might lose, it's so freeing. If I'm not really ok with it, I might choose to change more strategically and slowly. At this stage in my life, it's too painful (often physically) not to change when I get the nudge or inspiration.

Listening to my intuition, inspiration, higher self, higher power, God, the universe, source - whatever you choose to call your divine connection to all that is - is what I choose. Choice is just choice. And when I release judgment and don't label my choices good-bad, black-white, right-wrong, it's helpful. Then I'm free to just see what is more clearly and carry on with my quest for what's next, what's aligned, inspiring, even more fabulous, and feels like the right dynamic balance in this chapter of my life.

Sometimes, I have moments of incredible spaciousness, gazing at the water in awe of where I am and how happy I am. Other times, it's full on. To stay balanced, I imagine myself lightly skipping from rock to rock, making it across the stream without falling in. Sometimes, it's a super-fast flow, and I pretend I'm surfing and go with it. A form of spaciousness for me, is being "anchored up". If I'm not on a boat, I can still feel it. Quiet, still, curled up with a book and cocoa - waiting on what's next or letting the storm pass by.

As one of my friends once reminded me, "It's not all flow, all the time". Or, perhaps it's just a type of flow where it all works, just not always according to my immediate desire or preference. The flow may not be under my control (and for sure I count on myself, others, and the universe to deliver the results) … yet I know each state, step and moment, is mine to choose. Even if the choice is to let go and surrender. That's not a choice to give up. Just to do my best, let go, and send what's not working to the light.

You might be thinking, "That's all fine for you to say, but I'm different". I get it, you are. It's true. Your way of reaching for fabulous will be different. Your tools, spirit, speed, style, strategy, spirit, unique success - you'll keep evolving. Whatever works.

I get that changing sometimes feels out of reach. Or impossible. Have you ever felt that once you commit to the possibility that your choices create your experience, you're kind of stuck being responsible? That you lose your excuses? If you're like me and my clients, you're dancing on your growth edge, using all your tools and calling on spirit, and friends, and luck and your mind, heart, body and soul, and anything else that works to keep you dynamically balancing.

The growth edge represents opportunity, but it can sure feel sharp. If we're lucky, we just end up laughing at our humanness, bringing in some lightness. More amusing than spinning, spiraling or getting stuck down in "it".

When my state of being is somewhat less than fabulous, I remind myself that I get to choose. Or one of my friends does! By now, I know I can't control results - and certainly not other people. It's pretty simple. I get to choose not to react or fall into any old patterns or defaults that seriously don't work for me anymore. Actually, they never did. I notice the contrast, acknowledge what isn't working and pause in the moment.

The pause offers the spaciousness to respond or act, to discern what type of fab to reach for, and to sense what's next. It's all choice. Or rather, active choosing. Balance is never static and I'm open to new perspectives and possibilities. It's pretty magical having infinite possibilities at all times. I rarely worry about the opportunities that aren't showing up at present. I focus on mocking up what might be amazing, or something even better.

When I require a reminder to just do my fabulous best and then let go, I just remember the Serenity Prayer. God, grant me the Serenity to accept the things I can not change, the Courage to change the things I can, and the Wisdom to know the difference. It took me a long time to get that and live it. I'm still working on it. And no doubt always will be. It works.

As a woman, I've spent lots of time "trying" to be overly "on" and "doing it all". I spent a lot of time going for what I wanted on one hand and suppressing other aspects that were essential. I maxed out doing a lot of what I thought I had to do to get results in all areas of my life. Over and over. I still lean into my vision and actively pursue my desired outcomes; I just do it differently. Experiences, time, age, practice, deep trust, gratitude, meaningful work, creative expression, loving relationships, showing up as is, clarity about what matters most - it all plays into how I am being and creating now.

I've 98% ditched the perfectionist, do-it-all, "strive for superwoman" people-pleasing practice of my younger years. I highly recommend giving up what no longer serves you - sooner rather than later! My girlfriends too are embracing "if not now, when?!" So, it's now. We're all in that place. Find what works. Do it. Let go of the past. The failures (aka. learning experiences). Let go of the fear and drama (including our own), release OPEE (other people's emotions and expectations). Feel into and focus on what works. We're imperfectly focusing on what we want to create. I highly recommend this. Let's get clear, claim our brilliance, express our fabulosity, and illuminate what's possible.

Let's say you're listening to your calling, following your stars, your intuition, or your gut, but the right path isn't quite clear. Or maybe you're on a roll (or roller coaster!) and you're ready to reach for your next level - it might be even better than what you can imagine now! I've lightly touched on 3 power practices that work so consistently and effectively that I've integrated them into all that I do. (If you want my version, just reach out.) In the meantime, the beauty is that anyone can use their own tools, beliefs, and practices to implement these and experience their own results.

When I ask people what they want, even transformational leaders often rapidly respond with what they don't want. So, the question is what do you really, truly, deeply desire?

Notice what doesn't work, jot it down, and switch into imagining "What if I could?" and design for that or something even better. If you can't find your way, there's counseling, healing modalities or pick any activity (from being in nature or in your creative groove to doing the dishes) that really shifts your state so you're back to being you - glorious, grounded, centered, and ready. That's one way to let contrast guide you.

Or Shift into your power place and connect to your fabulous essence, higher self, God, mother, creator, source, all that is, the universe, spirit, your guides, your intuition, whatever you your words may be. Luxuriate in the spaciousness of connection. Allow answers to come and magic to happen. Maybe feel into your most fabulous future. You can dance lightly, let your imagination soar, be in your success frequency, and free to dream - all the way from inspiration to an inkling of an idea and even onwards to a strategically inspired action map.

Doing your energetic work is magical and practical too. It saves a ton of time, energy, stress, money… never mind enriching relationships, saying goodbye to negative interference, shoulda, woulda, coulda's, and lightening the load of day-to-day demands.

As I shift into my next chapter, my intention is to embrace create-ing and manifesting ever more lightly, focusing on the journey, allowing joy to bubble up, centering into what's genuine for me, and staying curious about what I'm not yet glimpsing. As usual, I'm committing to flow over hustle (even when it's fast flow!). I trust in what is coming, even though I don't know all the details and even when results differ from my expectations. Somehow, with enough time and realigning with what works fabulously, life always turns out beyond what I imagined. And so it is.

"It's a wrap!" - overheard on 1000s of photo shoots back in the day. I leave you with a small snapshot of what may come. My wish is for you, too, to delightedly and lightly follow your soul path with love, creativity, and adventure. You are a magical creative being with the intrinsic ability to design an amazing life. Trust yourself, fine-tune what works for you, and work it. Life is magical. Let's enjoy the journey together.

About Dinny Lansdowne

A creative entrepreneur, business advisor, and mentor to CSR and transformational businesses, Dinny's passion is to live fully, creatively, and - like the entrepreneurs she loves to work with - to be ever-evolving while having a meaningful impact and creating positive change. As a mentor, her joy and expertise is in helping change-makers make their visions come true. Dinny was the designer and CEO of a pioneering eco-social responsible designer clothing company, retailing and wholesaling her signature brands in her own boutique and across Canada and the USA. Since launching her agency, Inspired Source Media Inc., Dinny's clientele has included conscious business founders and their teams including Global Excellerated Business School, Retreat Guru, Visionary Hearts, as well as spiritually-guided wellness professionals and executives in leading-edge coaching and education. Her Fast Flow Mentoring integrates both the energetic and pragmatic aspects that empower conscious creators to transform not only their professional and business lives but also to align personally on all levels. To experience the 3 Power Practices, please visit inspiredmentors.com.

Chapter Nine

The Key to Navigating 50 is Self-Care, and I Help People Through Movement, Bodywork and Eventually...Acupuncture and Oriental Medicine!

by Lahela Hekekia

Sandy, at 91, walks everywhere (unaided) and does Pilates with me twice per week, as well as her home exercises, gets Acupuncture, reads, gardens, and paints. And she's very sharp of mind. I can't help but think that all that self-care promotes longevity. In our sessions, we concentrate on standing tall, balance, and flexibility. But this is huge: Sandy can get down to the floor and up again. She said, "I can do it because I do it every day. I have to do it every day." Simple yet profound guidance for a healthy life.

Well, if you currently find it challenging to get down to the floor and up again, there are ways to work towards it, including simple exercises. Sometimes, Physical Therapy is needed. Maybe it's not going to happen because of a physical issue. That's okay. We tailor the exercises to the individual. You can work on other things that are functional. If you do something every day, even 15 minutes of truly mindful breathing, you will be amazed at the impact on your life. Just breathing? Yes. Just breathing.

And did you know? Better posture really does improve breathing. There are many schools of thought in Pilates about proper breathing. I have my own approach, and I really like to emphasize specific ways of breathing while doing the spine work. And that's specifically because breathing IS spine work. I explain this in detail in solo and group sessions.

Would you be surprised to know that a large percentage of Pilates Teachers and Clients are women 40 and over? It is true! I endured chronic pain from ages 19-37, found Pilates, and never looked back. Everything else I do is complementary. But if you thought that Pilates was only for Ballerinas or youngsters, I have some great news for you!

That's Right… The Average Pilates Person is 40+, and many of us are 50+

In other words, you'll likely be in good company at the studio with people who understand what you're going through in terms of navigating 50 and beyond. I have been teaching Pilates since 2007 and doing Bodywork since 2001. My client base includes men and women up to age 91. (Did she just say 91? Yes, indeed!). As a Pilates Instructor, I have a number of clients who have started in their 70s and 80s and kept doing Pilates for years, even into their 90s. There's a modification for just about everyone in Pilates – and I've seen people literally transform themselves over time, even after traumatic incidents like strokes, spinal cord injuries, and brain surgeries.

Yes, Change IS Possible!

I continually witness people of all ages, sizes, and levels of fitness feel so much better in their bodies by improving their spine health, functional movement, and proprioception (the sense of: Where am I in space?). That is the greatest gift of Pilates, in my personal and professional opinion. I cannot speak for other Pilates teachers; this is what I do:

1. Analyze a person's posture and movement patterns, including gait (walking).

2. Ask them if they have any pain or any specific wellness goals.

3. Come up with a tailored workout that helps to address these concerns and goals.

4. Observe the client as they do the exercises.

5. Have a dialogue so that we become aware of the things that we observe.

6. Explain how to find the center of gravity and feel it in their body.

After a while, clients are correcting their own posture while sitting at the computer, standing in line at the grocery store, and going for a walk.

So, if someone were to ask if Pilates could help them navigate through bodily changes at 40, 50, and onward, I'd say absolutely. The better your posture, the better you can fill your lungs, and vice-versa. As neck, shoulder, and back tension decrease, and as breathing improves, this can go a long way in helping you feel more energetic. As joint and muscle balance improves, it can help you feel better taking a flight of stairs and enjoy your favorite sports and other physical activities. I used to be in chronic pain at 25, slouched over a computer for 16 hours a day. I don't have that discomfort any longer. My goal is to help each person improve.

What truly impressed me about Pilates was the focus on centering in the line of gravity. When I found that center line and kept working on it, especially on the Reformer and Cadillac (professional Pilates equipment), I noticed a huge change in flexibility and, over the years, changed my spine, hips, and feet. Then, I started experimenting with other people. One time, I was in a movement class, and as we were doing some preliminary stretches while seated on the ground, the person next to me was straining. I adjusted his legs in the hip joints very slightly, aligned his ankles and feet, moved his arms to a different position, and tapped his chest. He lifted his heart, sat up tall, and said, "Aha!" He was no longer straining into the stretch.

That was fun. So, from that and many similar experiences, I will go on record to say that if we can align our joints better in gravity and relation to one another, they will work better for us, including better flexibility. A lot of people will comment that they just aren't as flexible or mobile as when they were much younger. Well... I cannot make promises or provide a timeline. Still, I can say that Pilates can really improve one's flexibility if your teacher is helping you with your alignment in various postures -- lying down, sitting up, standing, and (if the body permits it) kneeling, and on all fours. That is a great tool to help navigate the body through life. So long as we have breath, we have an opportunity to make some positive changes.

Another thing that I love about Pilates are the spine exercises and how they are done with such precision. Oh, I could go on about how my spine improved through VERY MODIFIED Pilates exercises. I tell clients that these spine exercises can help support spine health and help them stand up tall and walk tall as a Senior because we are training all sorts of little muscles that help hold the spine upright. My hope is that we can continue to hold our spines upright throughout our lives. We want to think about it at 50 to keep ourselves mobile at 70, 80, and 90. Actually, we should be thinking about this at 15 since teens today tend to spend so much time on electronic devices, which can wreak havoc on their posture and core muscles. Side note: I have long suspected that Gen Z and Gen Alpha will experience neck and back issues a lot earlier in life than their Gen X parents because of the technology. Yes, there are exercises to help address a forward slouch, and all the affected muscles and joints in the spine, hips, knees, etc. But I'd rather teach someone how NOT to slouch. So yes, come to Pilates, and bring your teen. I'll paraphrase my mom, who always said this when I was a kid: They'll thank me at 35. Improving spine health is a great way to support your body as you walk through life.

Time and again, I have also watched clients achieve better balance, including a client, Alan, who worked with me in his late 80s. He was a brilliant Engineer who would analyze the exercises and tell me what we were doing and what he was sensing. After a few weeks, he announced that he no longer feared falling down the stairs because he could feel his body in space – so that he could bend his knees, reach an arm out to grasp the railing or do something else to regain his balance if he started to slip. His daughter also called and said, "I don't know what you're doing with Dad – but he seems to be more mentally sharp these days." (That was a day). Balance becomes increasingly important as we age because it's well-documented that falls are the leading cause of injury, as well as injury-related death, for adults ages 65 years and older. Bone loss (Osteoporosis and Osteopenia) and muscle loss (Sarcopenia) are common as we age, and this increases the risk of a fracture, which could significantly impact your independence.

So, anything we can do to help balance is a good thing, and the best time to start is NOW. You could start looking online at studios and offerings, look at teacher bios, and see who and what resonates with you.   It could be some other movement discipline, of course – Yoga Asana, Tai Chi, Dance, etc. One of the things that I have always emphasized, regardless of a client's age and athletic level, is to tune proprioception finely. What is Proprioception in general? It's that part of your nervous system that tells you, Where Am I In Space and What Am I Doing? I teach people how to discern their movements and whether they are staying within that center line of gravity – whether they are shifting, twisting, etc. In a way, we are magnifying the perception of your movements. By the way, it's entirely reasonable to not be sure what you're feeling in the beginning – it's a skill to develop. If someone says, "You say I'm centered, but I feel like I'm shifting way to the left," I explain that their BRAIN is getting used to a new normal – that retraining muscles and movement patterns involve brainwork too. If someone says, "I just can't feel it at all," or if they mention that they fall a lot, I give them special exercises to help improve Proprioception and will also consider referrals to other professionals to see if there are any underlying causes.

At times, adjunct therapy is useful to help support a healthy body. Depending on the circumstances, I suggest a Chiropractor or Osteopath (for a spine issue), an Acupuncturist (for so many reasons), or a Physical Therapist (for injuries or other conditions that will not be addressed with Pilates alone). Speaking of PT, many women start noticing around 50 (or even earlier) that they are waking up several times per night to pee. This is not a "normal" thing that you have to endure, and there are often things you can do about it. I have found that Pilates profoundly affected my bladder health by gently conditioning the Pelvic Floor with strength and flexibility. But I do refer clients to specialists on this subject.

Pilates exercises can seem "hard" sometimes. I might purposely challenge you with an exercise. We focus on enjoying the process. And since you live in your body every moment, you might not see the improvements that I see from week to week and over the long term. I am here to remind you what you have already accomplished. And this part is important:

Let's Rephrase the Self-Talk to Positive:

Clients are so used to me rephrasing any sort of negative self-talk. Yes, I realize that we are often our own worst critics (you are probably not surprised to know that we hear a lot of this in the wellness world). But maybe we should try treating ourselves like we would a best friend. Like, instead of looking at the mirror and saying *Ugh* -- how about saying, "Hey, there, I love you; it's just time to change things up a little bit." If you do it enough times, it starts to stick...

Here are two words that I often will reframe if the circumstances are right:

"I CAN'T"

Yes, those words can be necessary to protect your health and safety. Before starting, I always ask if you have any health concerns. Vertigo? Post Knee Surgery? A breathing issue? Chronic Pain? Sports injuries? Got it. You'll be asked follow-up questions, and we will come up with appropriate exercises and modifications. We might need a clearance (such as if you are doing physical therapy). Remember being a youth and hearing "No Pain, No Gain" from fitness gurus? I have always thought that was reckless advice. If you are verifiably in pain, you're injuring yourself. And Pilates is NOT meant to cause pain. People turn to Pilates all the time to help prevent sports injuries and for light training after completing Physical Therapy.

I'm talking about NOT convincing yourself that you're somehow inept and unable to achieve something. I learned the biggest lesson during Pilates teacher training. Having Scoliosis, I had to find a way to control my movements in a different way. We repeatedly tried one exercise in training, and I got frustrated about my form. Nobody else in the room had a spine issue, and I felt like I was holding everyone back. I finally said, "Well, I have Scoliosis; I guess I can't do this; let's just move on." My Teacher Trainer, Jayme, saw deeply into me, and her approach worked. I was training to teach other people to move! She said:

"Tell yourself that you don't have Scoliosis."

"But I do have Scoliosis; I have the x-rays and everything," I replied.

"Just try telling yourself that you don't have it," she said.

"But ... I do!"

(This went on for a few minutes until the light bulb went on over my head)

"Wait... Oh! I don't have Scoliosis."

Then, I tried the exercise one more time and didn't focus on looking the same way as my fellow teachers-in-training. Later in the Teacher Training Program, we did the same exercise on a different piece of equipment – the Ladder Barrel -- and it went much better than on the Reformer. So, we found the optimal place for me to work on that exercise.

I finally understood Jayme's point. And it was probably the most important lesson from Pilates Teacher Training. I was focusing on the wrong outcome (instant perfection) and giving up. I also defined myself by a supposed limitation and did not even give myself time to work things through. I asked myself, how could I teach people to move if I had a self-defeating attitude? Recognizing an injury, a spine condition or some other challenge is necessary, but it's important to give ourselves empowering self-talk. This situation is really okay. If the movement is comfortable, we can keep working through it. Another amazing Pilates mentor, Pat, advised me to say, instead of some self-criticism:

"Well, that was interesting."

Also, that I had an "interesting leg," not a "bad leg." Words make a huge difference. And ever since then (2007), if an exercise is difficult, or if there is a challenge with balance, flexibility, or something else, I just remind clients to add one word that is truly empowering:

"I can't do that exercise ... YET."

I tell them this allows us to acknowledge challenges and yet leave the door open for future success. If we say, "I can't," then the Mind will say, "Fine, then let's not even try." And where the Mind goes, the Body will follow. But if we just leave that door open, the Mind will be open to trying some modifications, alternate exercises, or perhaps a detour and circling back later. I have worked with people who had challenges with coordinating movements after spine injuries, strokes, and brain surgeries, but with enough time, there was an improvement. I remind them all the time what they have achieved over the long term. I'm big on telling ourselves and each other that Change IS Possible. If we do something as simple and profound as changing our breathing and posture, these have an enormous impact. We do these things every day, all day – and changing that is truly Core work.

50 is Not a Downhill Slope -- We can look forward to ages 70-90.

Clients always inspire – and to be honest, they often navigate me!

When you see such spark, it makes you realize that this thing called Fifty is still YOUNG and is a great time to really invest in your well-being and enjoy it. Let me tell you about some amazing people in my life:

TBT: It's 2016 and in walks Hale (Pronounced "Hah-lay"). She was in her late 80s but could easily pass for much younger age. She moved so fluidly on the Reformer and Cadillac (professional Pilates equipment), and we worked together for years. A renowned Hula dancer who was taught by the true greats, Hale brought her Hula sister Likelike (Pronounced "Lee-kay Lee kay) for Pilates (who was in her 70s, but you'd never know it). We also worked together for years. Oh, they're still around, very sharp of mind, and lovely as ever. Things just changed due to the Pandemic, parent caregiving, and all sorts of things. Life goes on!

One day, I mentioned that I was getting married and that I wanted to do a Wedding Hula. Hale and Likelike volunteered to teach me and then did a surprise dress rehearsal by inviting me to a gathering of their Hula Sisters. Many of them were in their 80s and 90s, all of them just stunning singers and dancers, professional performers from the 1950s and 1960s. Hale was 90 at this point. I had no idea how the 1950s style of dancing Hula was so glamorous and full of humor; I had never seen anything like it. I was laughing and crying. There was one duet in which my friend's mother was singing the song in 'Olelo Hawai'i and playing her guitar. And her cohort was dancing in perfect sync while reciting the English translation. And she'd do a little wink to explain the hidden meaning of the song (because the Hawaiian language was traditionally multilayered). And I think I still have the video on my cell phone of Hale dancing so fluidly, with a gorgeous smile, and so sharp of mind (she still is). If the Universe wills me to make it to 80-90, I hope to be that graceful and full of energy. What Hale told me, as well, was that as their group of friends got older and their numbers grew smaller, the gatherings had gotten increasingly lively. They knew that tomorrow together was uncertain, so they were very much in the present with one another. Wow. Great advice.

As I'm in my reverie, watching the scene, Hale gets on the mic and says:

"Lahela, come on up here and dance."

"Huh?" (suddenly, my heart starts pounding).

Well, when your teacher says to get up and dance, you just do it. Hale and her friends jumped up too, and we danced my wedding Hula. And then of course, the ladies gathered around and gave hilarious marriage advice! And I will treasure that day, and their gift.

As I mentioned earlier, I will eventually be able to provide acupuncture and Oriental medicine. I'm currently working towards a Doctorate and see so many ways to help support and improve people's well-being. I have seen in Clinic people turning to Acupuncture for all sorts of things, including getting better sleep, improved immune function, and more. I am really drawn to Orthopedic Acupuncture and all the ways that it can help with injuries and chronic pain. I look forward to learning more.

About Lahela Hekekia

Lahela Hekekia is a Nationally Certified Pilates Teacher specializing in injuries, sports injury prevention, and spine issues such as Scoliosis. After getting certified through STOTT PILATES®, she found a Classical mentor, Pat Guyton, who is known around the world. Lahela also teaches people how to move more freely through Franklin Method®, and she is a Level III Certified Movement Educator. Lahela is, moreover, a Licensed Massage Therapist and a Certified Graston Technique® Specialist, working with clients with pain and injury. She has taught Massage Therapy courses, including Medical Myotherapy. Lahela looks forward to learning more at Acupuncture School and adding that to her list of offerings in the future. A lifelong resident of Hawaii, Lahela sees clients in Kailua, and Honolulu.

Chapter Ten
All Is In Divine Order
by Denise DeSimone

"There are two ways to live: You can live as if nothing is a miracle; or you can live as if everything is a miracle."

- Albert Einstein

B lessings in our lives come in all shapes, sizes, and forms at different times and in different ways.

It may sound odd, that the greatest gift of my life was being diagnosed with stage IV throat and neck cancer. I was one week away from my 50th birthday and they told me I may have only three months to live. Was it tough? Yes. Was it scary? Yes. Was it the most profound time of my life? Absolutely. Here is a snippet of the lessons I learned, especially the lessons learned regarding trusting the universe and knowing all is in Divine order.

Whatever life lays out for us we can always turn challenges into doorways of transformation. This is exactly what I did and continue to do with every challenge I face.

SEPTEMBER 2005

My prayer:

I am one with God's perfect wisdom of health! It's interesting that this area of my body, my throat and neck, is affected. The channel between body and mind or is the mind in the head. In any event, the center of communication is affected. And this is a time for me to connect with the highest vibration of communication, of source, of my life. I ask for deep forgiveness around all the ill thoughts. I release all fear around people knowing my secrets of the dark places in my life. I am not those dark places. I am the light of the world and God's love is my focus.

In the words of Gloria Gaynor:

I will survive.

I got all my life to live.

I got all my love to give.

I will survive.

Sleep didn't come easy. I tossed and turned while I wrestled with relentless thoughts of anxiety, fear, and sadness. When dawn finally arrived, I reached for the piece of paper with the woman's contact information from the health food store. Our meeting one another had not been by chance. My next step had already been revealed before I even knew I needed it. I had sensed she was the angel, sent by divine intervention, and was going to lead me into the hands of the medical team I now so desperately needed. I was anxious to dial her number, but telephoning a stranger this early in the day seemed too personal.

Because of my strong meditation practice, I was aware of the calming power of connecting to my breath, so while I waited to call her, I focused on slowing my breathing to help me remain calm.

At that moment, the telephone beside me rang. It was my dear friend Paula. She called to see how I was holding up. News of my biopsy had traveled fast, and Paula wasted no time in calling.

Paula and I met ten years ago at our church, Unity on The River.

Unity is a spiritual community that welcomes and honors all paths to God. It is a positive and practical philosophy that promotes a way of life that leads to health, prosperity, happiness, and peace of mind.

I was thankful I had a spiritual community like Unity on The River. I was also thankful I had built a strong spiritual foundation. And it was rocked.

Paula is a beautiful, dark-haired Italian woman with chestnut eyes and wavy dark hair. She is an artist in every sense of the word, from the poetic way in which she speaks, to the clothes she wears, layering her garments upon her body just as she layers paint on a canvas.

After a silence that was thick with emotion, Paula asked me if I would like to pray, and of course, I said yes.

Before she began the prayer, Paula softly whispered, "You didn't do anything wrong."

Her tender words soothed my wounded heart, and I began to sob. On some level, I knew what Paula had said was true, but I sure felt like I had done something wrong.

Too often we are scolded, not only as children, but as adults for doing something "wrong." I loathed the word "wrong." My spirit loathed the word "wrong."

We never do anything wrong. There is no wrong. There just is what is. No matter what I might have done in the past, when I chose to do what I did, it seemed like a good idea at the time. I had matured enough spiritually to know I created my own reality by what and how I thought, but since I never consciously chose this I must have done something wrong. It wasn't deliberate.

This situation grabbed me by the neck and rattled me to my core. My ego wanted to play with my head and destroy my spirit. My humanness flooded in, and the voice of Spirit was forced out. An acronym for EGO is, Edging God Out. I got sucked into Edging God Out.

Eckhart Tolle says in his book, A New Earth: The voice of the ego continuously disrupts the body's natural state of well-being. Almost every human body is under a great deal of strain and stress, not because it is threatened by some external factor but from within the mind. The body has an ego attached to it, and it cannot help but respond to all the dysfunctional thought patterns that make up the ego. Thus, a stream of negative emotion accompanies the stream of incessant and compulsive thinking.

I was an incessant and compulsive thinker.

I couldn't fully digest her message at that time but Paula's reassurance, "You didn't do anything wrong" eventually opened me to the process of finally looking at my clandestine guilt.

I didn't know it then but instead of beating myself up, I needed my spirituality to forgive my personality and allow for my humanness.

Then it was time for Paula and me to pray, time to trust the process and time to thank my ego for sharing. Centered prayers from the place of knowing that all is in divine order flowed through Paula and me; that place that knows only good, only love, only wholeness and only peace, oneness and light.

I told Paula about the woman at the health food store and that I was anxious to call her.

Paula said, "I hope she is someone who can help. I'll talk to you soon."

At eight o'clock. I dialed the number on the piece of paper and Alice answered the phone.

"Hello Alice?"

"Yes."

"My name is Denise DeSimone; I met you yesterday at the health…"

Before I could finish my opening sentence, Alice said, "I have been thinking about you since we met yesterday. How did it go?"

I took a deep breath, paused, and said, "It didn't turn out so well. I need to see an oncologist and I wonder if you could tell me a bit more about your doctor in Boston."

Alice was not only willing to share her medical reference, but she was also generous with her time, because from her own experience she knew what I was going through and spent the better part of an hour on the phone with me.

The team of doctors she recommended at Massachusetts Eye and Ear Infirmary were the premier physicians in the field of head and neck oncology. People from all over the world seek treatment from these teams. Should I encounter any delays in setting an appointment, Alice offered to help.

The word oncology didn't freak me out quite as much that day as it did the day before because now it had a "they can save my life" kind of ring to it.

There is nothing quite like a cancer diagnosis to help prioritize your life. Things that seemed so critical just yesterday; like my daily routine, going to church, making sure I was well put together before heading out the door and eating all the right things, now paled in comparison. But I needed to begin this day as normally as possible, so I took myself for a walk to help clear my head before making that emotional phone call to the Boston doctors.

For the next few days, I was in slow motion. I did not have the emotional energy to move forward at my normal rapid-fire speed. Yet, at the same time, I couldn't devour life fast enough. To say I was devastated was an understatement. What could possibly be the reason for being served a death sentence?

I felt exposed in an unfamiliar way, turned inside out, tender, and immobilized by it all. My eyes were constantly misty, not just because I was sad, but because life was so precious and may be cut short. Looking deeply into the eyes of those I loved, I wondered if those moments were some of the last moments we would share. I was vulnerable. Vulnerability was the only "ability" I possessed.

I wanted to reach out through my vulnerability to my family, my friends and my spiritual community and invite them into my process. I needed their love and support. I didn't want to go through this challenging time alone. Being single and having no children left space for me to create my family of choice.

For several years I had been emailing daily messages of inspiration to a handful of friends and family. I called this "The Daily Dose." What had started with just a few people had now grown to nearly 60 recipients. This was the perfect vehicle for sharing my sad news.

"The Daily Dose"

September 5, 2005

Dear friends,

I had to go in for surgery to remove a few swollen lymph nodes that didn't have the courtesy to return to their normal size on their own. Well, things turned out a bit differently than we thought they would. Some nasty little cells found their way into my space and now we need to help them find their way out.

I am fortunate in that I have an appointment to see one of the best doctors and his team at Mass Eye and Ear in Boston. Next Thursday I will talk with these folks and set a plan of action into place. The next few days/weeks/hopefully not months might be a bit challenging to me and my request is that you keep the high watch for me.

Love is a painkiller, and you are all filled with such love that I just know I will be fine, and any pain will be at a minimum. Together we can move mountains so...I know we can usher these cells on their way. There may be times when the Daily Dose will have some gaps and at those times know that God and I are doing all we can to return to sending out the Daily Dose. One of my most precious moments of each day, is connecting with each of you.

Healthfully yours,
Denise

Almost immediately, my inbox was busy with well wishes and heartfelt concerns from the Daily Dose recipients. They comforted me and told me they would keep me at the top of their prayer list.

The bitterness of this cancer diagnosis had been soothed by the sweetness of their love for me. Tremendous surges of love bathed me energetically to where I needed to manage it. Managing love's tidal waves, I pictured those tiny, red, Valentine's Day candied hearts, as they melted into my being, each one saturated one cell at a time, filling me with light and love, until my entire body was warm from the imaginary heat of these liquefied hearts. This exercise had helped me use their love in a tangible way.

Before I was diagnosed, I had doubted the love of my family and friends. On the surface, sure, I knew I was loved. However, my deeper self, the wounded self, felt unloved.

Clearly, I was loved. Family and friends poured their love all over me in so many ways. There was something to loving myself that had to do with healing myself. This was an area that was going to require deeper insight. It took me a while to realize it was the lack of self-love that had been the missing link.

I needed the catharsis of journaling. I transferred thoughts to words. I allowed my unedited feelings to flow from my heart and onto the paper. I felt the freedom to oust my emotions, to let them spill over onto the pages as I released the sadness from the depths of my being.

The new journal I had purchased specifically for this journey held such generosity in the quality of the paper. The pen would sink into the fiber just enough to return exactly what I needed to remain present to the process.

I had to trust the process, and I needed to trust God. At the same time, I knew I needed to allow for my humanness. I needed to feel all of it.

Time to pray:

Dear God,

I know I am being held at this time. Together we will see me through this challenge with strength, gentleness and most of all love. I see my body strong and healthy, knowing there are more healthy cells than there are dis-eased. I will sing myself to wholeness, laugh myself to health and breathe myself into balance.

I am granted peace and joy and good health all these days moving toward my birthday and beyond. I am grateful in advance for the fun, laughter, kindness and my good strong dancing body during my 50th birthday celebration. I hold my family and friends in joy and love for this I am forever grateful.

When I went to see the oncologists in Boston to whom I had been referred, they said they did not have enough information and we needed further testing. I was happy the necessary tests were scheduled for after my birthday celebration.

It was time for another update.

Dear hearts,

Thank you all for your well wishes, prayers and love.

Next week on Monday and Tuesday I will be in Mass Eye and Ear going through several tests. Friday, I meet with a team of treatment doctors and set the stage for what will be the most difficult ride of my life.

On the physical plane this is a very serious situation and on the spiritual level this is an opportunity for us to hold the highest vibration we can muster. To say I am not scared would be a lie. I am very scared. And I will choose faith over fear. I am truly grounded in my faith, in my belief that all things are for a higher and greater purpose, more than anything…love always prevails.

I am so blessed with the people in my life. There are no words to describe the depths to which I feel this connection. In the face of all that is going on, I feel like I am the wealthiest woman on the planet. Because when it comes right down to it...all we really have is each other.

Thank you for holding me close. Love yourselves unconditionally. You are my medicine!

Love,
Denise

An email tsunami flooded my inbox with an outpouring of affection from many considerate and loving souls. It felt like Christmas in September.

How could I have ever doubted the love of my friends and family? I truly did feel like the wealthiest woman on the planet.

So many people equate wealth with money. I realized I could have been more successful financially. I could have developed a more serious career and acquired huge assets. In the final analysis of my place in life, I had developed a career. I had developed a career out of loving people. These people were my markers for success. My wealth had nothing to do with money. It had everything to do with love, connection, and experience of the rich and raw healing power of love.

There's a Tim McGraw song about a man who receives a cancer diagnosis, and a friend asks, "So what did you do when they told you the bad news?" The man's response,; "I went sky diving, I went Rocky Mountain climbing, I went 2.7 seconds on a bull named Fu Man Chu, and I loved deeper, and I spoke sweeter, and I gave forgiveness I'd been denying. Some day I hope you get the chance to live like you were dying."

I had related to this at a visceral level.

Every cell of my being had been permeated with gratitude for having been granted this opportunity to live like I was dying. I would walk around my house singing the words to that song so loudly, I was sure the mere vibration of my voice would shake the cancer loose.

The strange paradox: I would never ever wish a diagnosis of cancer on anyone, yet...at the same time... if only for one day, I had wished others could participate in life at this level.

About Denise DeSimone

AUTHOR, SPEAKER, SPIRITUAL MENTOR, PODCASTER, DOCUMENTARIAN, INTERFAITH MINISTER.

Denise DeSimone is a sought-after inspirational speaker and teacher who travels the country sharing her mission and message of inspiration as a "thriver" of stage IV throat and neck cancer. Denise is also a spiritual mentor for cancer patients and others helping them to turn challenges into doorways of transformation.

Denise's book, FROM STAGE IV TO CENTER STAGE as well as her documentary by the same name have inspired thousands worldwide. Denise's purpose in life is to enjoy. Her mission is to compassionately spread joy and encourage laughter. Her vision is, that all sentient beings know the peaceful power of self-love.

In 2015, her love for her beloved Italy encouraged her to start a boutique travel company taking small groups, (spring & fall) to tour her village of Paciano, Italy and many villages of Tuscany.

Website: www.denisedesimone.com

Email: denise@denisedesimone.com

Cell: 978-407-8107

Chapter Eleven

The Life I Imagine: Creating Reality from The Heart

by Catherine Stilo

B oldly staring back from the cover of a journal I fished out of my bottom drawer is a quote by Henry David Thoreau:

"Go confidently in the direction of your dreams! Live the life you've imagined."

I received this journal as a gift almost two decades ago. Feeling it was too precious to write in, I had actually forgotten about it until I went in search of a notebook to collect my inspirations. I felt the cosmic humor, the Universe chuckling, already knowing what I was going to write and providing the thread to tie it together.

I remember a moment in a Plant Medicine Ceremony, one of the Shamans waving feathers in a smoke-clearing ritual, saying, "Focus on you. Focus only on you, only your own energy. Just you. Just you." In the chaos of all the energies, it wasn't easy. After over half a century on this planet, much training and teaching, I still felt challenged to focus only on ME, and it wasn't just this moment in Ceremony. This moment revealed a broader pattern in life.

I realized that "ME" was buried beneath layers of expectations, masks I had chosen to conform to what others valued or what I interpreted as being valued. I had gotten tangled up in other people's feelings, energies, and expectations. How I do things, what I really love, my true offerings, and my true gifts to the world got set aside and forgotten in that bottom drawer. Noticing this, I started asking, "Who am I? Who do I want to be? What vibration do I want to hold?" If I chose one way, surely I could choose another?

This choice gets complicated because sometimes the voices I think belong to others are actually my own expectations projected outward and reflected back. I blame others for what is only my own reflection. For me, this happens with PERFECTIONISTIC tendencies – my own judgment of my work and lack of self-compassion is in the way of full expression of being, even though, at times, it takes the form of other faces. I project those tendencies out onto someone or something external, and they stare back at me in a way that allows me to learn something about myself.

Sometimes, I think I have transcended expectations, and other things, like old wounds, resurface. My 8-year-old self shows up replaying stories of hurt, exclusion, and rejection. Those patterns don't always disappear after the memory fades. Those same patterns continue to impact my adult interactions until I learn the lesson.

When I received the invitation to write a chapter in this book, my first instinct was to jump on the opportunity immediately based only on a "vibe." I hesitated acting on impulse, because an old wound that resulted in a very hard and painful lesson eerily resembled this same opportunity. To untangle myself from its grip, I needed to understand the energy I brought and how I contributed to the dynamic of the situation; otherwise, I would risk tripping again. If I got stuck in that pattern or believed because it happened once, it will happen again, I would miss an opportunity and continue to replicate that story.

Complicating things even further, sometimes, the wounds aren't even my own. They are steeped in lineage as I witness myself repeating parental patterns, turning out "just like my parents." In my hesitation after almost impulsively acting, I spiraled down a rabbit hole of story. This opportunity seemed so good, almost too good to be true, that I had to back-fill what was wrong with it. I dove deep, spinning a story of "bait and switch" where after initial agreement comes commitment that hadn't been disclosed. The emotion I created by weaving stories was incredibly intense. With a simple phone call, everything was clarified. None of my stories proved true but the emotion remained so strong, I wanted to continue to believe what I made up.

Now, the irony is that I spiraled down that rabbit hole, having just watched my father, Frank, do exactly the same thing with another situation only a day earlier. In an instant, I became both extremely compassionate for my father and extremely concerned for myself at this apparently inherited pattern. Is it possible this story is rooted somewhere in my lineage? Here I am, essentially with a dream handed to me, always having wanted to be an author, having had many inspirations for a book and what am I doing? I had to laugh out loud when my partner pointed out, "Wow, you really 'Franked' the s#@! out of that one!" Sometimes, the generational chasm that I think is miles-wide is actually only a few inches.

Why do I cling to those old stories and wounds? I had a vision so profound, again in Ceremony, when I asked, "Why can't I let go of the things holding me back? Why is it so challenging to move forward even when I have a deep desire?" A vision came to me of my own hands, cupped together, holding something. Peeking inside, I saw a small crumpled piece of white paper and a voice defended "MINE!". The image was reminiscent of the character "Gollum" in The Lord of the Rings declaring "my Precious" while clutching the One Ring. The paper is the story or identity I hold of who I am. I am holding this so tightly and defining myself so tightly in this way that my hands are cramped shut with no way of letting it go and no room to let anything else in. The symbolism of the crumpled paper for me is that it's garbage. It's something that should have been thrown out, but I can't. So why can't I?

When I first answered that question, I said "FEAR"; however, that answer felt incomplete. I need to understand the root of the fear.

Whatever the story, whatever is written on that piece of paper...be it my "smallness," "not worthy," or the opposite "title or achievement," or "what I do for a living,"...it is some way I define myself. If I let go, it means letting go of an idea on which I have built my entire identity - "My Precious." Even my own pain defines me. It's everything I have built myself on. If I let go, how will I know who to be?

Looping back to my own perfectionistic tendencies, the funny thing is, those tendencies have also been my greatest advantage. Those tendencies fueled me to achieve in many areas, led me never to be satisfied, always wanting to be better. Whether it be in work, fitness, relationships, those tendencies are both the drivers and the deterrents. The key is to learn to channel those tendencies to propel me forward.

That momentum starts by saying "YES" to doing something I love, but it doesn't get easy from there. Putting myself out there stirs things up. Taking action brings me face-to-face with my shadow. Saying "YES" is the beginning of an ego match with the small self. Here's a ringside seat to my "main event."

"I don't have anything to say. I'm not a writer." Oh my goodness! Out of nowhere! A left jab from ego. The reality is I've had so many ideas and inspirations over the years. I never wrote because Ego's story then was, "There's no point. It's a waste of time. There are so many more important things to do." The point being that I love to write. It is fun. The concept of doing things just for pleasure was so foreign, though, that I didn't.

The ego is relentless and keeps pressing forward with a flying knee. "The problem isn't not enough to say, it's that you have too much to say." (The ego switches to second person, talking at me, not as me.) "Your ideas are all over the place. You have too much, and you don't know how to organize it."

As so often happens, a solution appears. In a brief chat with Betsy Chasse (the publisher), she gave an example of another story in the book and framed the idea in the form of a question. Ah! Right. Frame my idea in the form of a question, write down all the inspirations, and re-organize them, discarding anything that wanders from the thread to answer the question. Problem solved.

Immediately after hanging up, trying to close out the win, ego with a wheel-kick to the head:

"OMG. I don't have a story. What was I thinking? That story is profound. That story makes a difference. What do I know? I'm not a [profession]. My story is nowhere near as good! It's drivel." I almost bowed out, comparing the story I hadn't even written to one I hadn't even read.

Oh, she's down! She's hurt!

The Ego, knowing with a good shot, she'll be out, jumps right in with an aggressive left hook on top and a knife right to the body – the threat and consequence.

"This is your first published work. If you put it out there and, it's s!@#, YOUR CAREER AS AN AUTHOR WILL BE RUINED! YOU'LL NEVER GET ANOTHER CHANCE! NO ONE WILL WANT TO LISTEN TO YOU!"

And then, one last hit, the knock-out punch, the lowest blow of all after the first draft…

"What a pedantic, self-indulgent showpiece. NO ONE wants to hear your story. There is no reason to even submit it."

There is something to be said about sitting on dreams. If I don't do anything, in my head, I can always be a brilliant writer. Pen to paper opens another possible truth, but does it matter? The point isn't achieving greatness; it's the love of the process.

So, the key to overcoming programming, old wounds, inherited traits, and the ego match with the small self? I go into my heart and listen for that quiet voice of intuition. Here's how I get there:

Move! Get more fluid! Make movement enjoyable. Let go of ideas of "should" and listen to what the body needs to bring balance—maybe a quiet, gentler practice or a vigorous one to shake things up. If I become too rigid in my practices, even the thing I love can become the thing I loathe because I am forcing myself to do it without honoring my body or at a time in disharmony with natural rhythms.

Dance it out! As a die-hard Grey's Anatomy fan, I know Shonda Rhimes was on to something. As I began to learn about the fascia in the body and somatic practices, I began to experience first-hand that these stories and wounds reside locked in the tissues and can be released with movement. Moving the body softens the physical patterns of constriction and enhances the flow of energy.

Go into Nature! Find "Beauty Moments," moments of grateful awe at the magnificence of this world. It might be a long, vigorous hike, or it might simply be a moment to sit and observe. It was challenging at first, but once I started, "Beauty Moments" became exponential, and I began seeing beauty in all of life, including its lessons.

Meditate! But beyond conventional ways. I let go of the notion of sitting uncomfortably in lotus position for hours, fighting the chatter of the mind and chastising myself for never actually achieving what I set out to achieve. I replaced the idea of eliminating mind chatter with the idea of turning down the volume on the chatter and up the volume on the Voice of Spirit. I invited pleasure in. When I started to look at meditation as pleasure or pleasure as meditation, things shifted. I started to go for the feeling being generated, not holding on to a story about the form. Sitting with a coffee cup at sunrise, maybe it's only 3 minutes before the rest of the house gets up...1 minute...30 seconds...one breath all can be moments where there is an influx of Spirit, and I'm connected with everything and everyone. Meditation is not an end in itself, a checkmark on my "to-do" list. It's a bridge to Spirit, to open myself to my own voice of intuition. With consistent practice, I started to hear it.

What does this Voice of Spirit sound like? It's a whisper I hear when I quiet the chatter and rise above the drama. This whisper is so quiet, a very faint "Hey!" often coming just as I open my eyes in the morning or while doing mundane tasks during the day.

Distinguishing between Spirit and the ego jumping in took practice. Spirit's voice is a whisper, maybe conversational level at best, no louder, mostly a whisper so quiet I have to say "What? What was that?" and strain to hear. It's also very simple—one word, two words, or a burst of inspiration without words, a feeling but without emotional charge. It's very calm, neutral and holds no expectations either way, whether I follow or not.

On the other hand, the ego's voice is SUPER LOUD. Imagine writing a text. Ego comes ALL IN CAPS, yelling and very chatty. There's a lot of very rapid Blah! Blah, blah, blah, blah! So much that I don't even know what the f@#$ it is saying because there is way too much information. It is also super-charged and throws in consequences…if you don't do this, you're going to be THWAA! (sound of dire outcome) or if you do this, you're going to be YEAAAAAAH! (sound of celebration). That's exactly what it sounds like.

And once I hear it…listen to it. Follow and re-follow it. I know my choices determine the vibration I put into the world, and that vibration ultimately creates the world I experience. I know I live the life I imagine. The world responds to the beliefs I have buried deep inside. Feelings paint pictures and build worlds. I just need to make absolutely sure those imaginings are the whispers of my own heart, not ones I have been fed, bought into, or have stuck on repeat.

Do I go confidently in the direction of my dreams? LOL! At least I have fished them out of that bottom drawer and got myself pointed the right way!

About Catherine Stilo

Drawing from over three decades of personal study and training and a passion for movement, Catherine creatively blends yogic teaching and sensory awareness with the art of story and a deep connection to the natural world.

In 2013, she embarked on an adventure to live a life in greater harmony with herself and with natural rhythms. That journey led to some amazing places, events, and experiences.

She is an Experienced Yoga Teacher recognized with Yoga Alliance (E-RYT 500), holds certifications in Group Fitness (American Council on Exercise) and Permaculture Design (Whole Systems Design LLC.), and continually explores both mainstream and esoteric philosophies and teachings.

Her mission is to share the magic of feeling wildly alive, fully embodied, and living a more authentic, connected life. When not teaching or training, you'll find her barefoot in the grass, flowing with the peaceful, alive, and "unplugged" vibes.

Visit TerraKula.org to find out more about her adventures and upcoming workshops.

Chapter Twelve

Shake It Off: Biohacking Health, Hormones, and Happiness

by Lisa Dimond

Have you ever noticed that hitting our 50s and beyond feels like we've been issued an official "Welcome to the Golden Girls Club"?

Our skin loses its bounce, wrinkles stage a hostile takeover, and our memory becomes more like a faulty GPS. Metabolism? Let's just say it's seen better days. And for women, there's the joyride known as menopause.

This "I'm getting old syndrome" sneaks into every nook and cranny of our lives—relationships, careers, even our personal joy. It chips away at our confidence, pokes at our self-esteem, throws a wet blanket on our libido, siphons our energy, and turns our motivation into a couch potato. Sleep? Focus? Overall zest for life? All on the fritz.

Mainstream advice? Pop pills, inject Botox, and go under the knife. Society keeps chanting that aging is a war zone and Father Time is the enemy.

But here's the kicker: that's yesterday's news. It's outdated and honestly, not even in the realm of what's truly possible.

Ladies let's talk about a little secret that's been buzzing around the fitness world (actually, for decades) – and no, it's not the latest diet fad or some miracle pill. It's something far more exciting and backed by science. We're diving into the world of Whole Body Vibration (WBV), a groundbreaking approach to health and wellness that's particularly beneficial for women at any age but especially those in their fabulous fifties. Imagine standing on a platform, letting it gently vibrate your worries (and calories) away. Sounds intriguing? It sure does!

You may remember the very funny scene from "I Love Lucy", using the vibrating belt machine at the gym. My earliest memory of vibration was at the age of 4 or 5. I would accompany my grandmother, Nannie, to the Elaine Powers Figure Salon. No childcare in fitness centers back then, so I would follow her from one piece of equipment to the other. My favorite - the vibrating belt. I would place my tiny little hand on the side of her leg just below her hip to feel the good vibes. I remember feeling so happy and delighted. Roughly 38 years later, I would once again feel vibration in a fitness setting and never look back. I was reintroduced to Whole Body Vibration and specifically Power Plate in 2008. A short five years later, I founded BVibrant - A Powerful Health & Wellness Studio in Naples, FL and became a Master Trainer. When someone would ask me what I do for a living, I would respond with, "I have the largest vibrator in town and help people achieve optimal health and fitness".

Vibration therapy has come a long way since the vibrating belts of the 1950s and 60s. To understand its benefits today, let's take a quick trip through its history.

Vibration therapy dates back to Ancient Greece and Rome, where it was used to heal wounded warriors. Without modern technology, they mimicked the effects through activities like sawing wood, plucking large instruments, and horseback riding.

In the 18th century, three key figures revolutionized vibration therapy. In France, Jean-Martin Charcot explored how vibrations from train and carriage rides alleviated Parkinson's symptoms. He even invented a chair to replicate these vibrations. Meanwhile, in Sweden, Gustav Zander, a gym pioneer, created exercise machines that used vibrations to boost weight loss and muscle mass. In the U.S., Dr. John Harvey Kellogg, better known for Corn Flakes, developed steam-powered vibration chairs and platforms for his Battle Creek Sanatorium.

Jump to the 1960s, when German scientists developed rhythmic neuromuscular stimulation, and Russian Olympic teams used whole-body vibration (WBV) machines to great success, winning a record number of medals in 1960. By the mid-1990s, WBV had made its way to space, with Russian cosmonauts using it to combat muscle atrophy and improve bone density, leading to a record 438 days in space. NASA soon followed suit.

To date, over 20,000 research studies have been published on Whole Body Vibration. In recent years most of the research is conducted on Power Plates. As Nikola Tesla said, "If you want to find the secrets of the universe, think in terms of energy, frequency, and vibration." The same applies to health and wellness. WBV can help you biohack your health, hormones, and happiness well beyond age 50.

As we gracefully glide through our 40s, 50s, and beyond, maintaining our health becomes a top priority. Whether it's keeping our bones strong, muscles toned, or simply ensuring our overall well-being, WBV offers an innovative and enjoyable way to achieve these goals and you don't have to spend hours in the gym. So, let's shake things up and explore how this magical platform can make a difference in our lives.

Before we dive into the benefits, let's get acquainted with what WBV actually is. Picture this: a sleek platform that vibrates at various frequencies. When you stand, sit, or even exercise on it, these vibrations are transmitted through your body, stimulating muscles, tendons, and bones in ways traditional workouts might not. The plate, and I'm specifically referring to Power Plate (which uses a patented PrecisionWave™ Technology), is vibrating in three directions: forward-backward, up and down, and side-to-side, almost simultaneously. This movement, known as Tri-Planar vibration, creates a reflex response in the body. The multi-dimensional movement creates a harmonic vibration and depending on the level of frequency set, the harmonic vibration in turn creates involuntary muscle contractions. So, if the plate is set at a frequency of 30hz, you will experience 30 contractions per second. In a traditional gym setting, you may experience 1-2 contractions per second.

The body's reflexes are going to naturally cause the nervous system to respond and stimulate these systems in the body: neurological, proprioceptive, musculoskeletal, cardiovascular, hormonal. When these systems are activated you will see benefits like quicker fat burning, tighter skin, stronger muscles, improved flexibility, more core strength, increased circulation, stronger bones.

So, what makes WBV the darling of the fitness world, especially for women in their fabulous 50s and beyond? Let's explore the top four areas of structure, circulation, metabolism and hormones that benefit from vibration therapy, backed by solid research and science.

Your Structural Foundation Is Your Fountain of Youth.

Bone Health: Let's face it – bone health becomes a significant concern as we age, particularly post-menopause. With the decline in estrogen levels, our bones can become more fragile, making us more susceptible to osteoporosis and fractures. Enter WBV, our new best friend in the fight against bone density loss.

Research shows that WBV can significantly enhance bone density. A study published in the Journal of Bone and Mineral Research found that WBV increased bone formation markers in postmenopausal women. The vibrations stimulate bone cells, promoting growth and strength, much like how weight-bearing exercises do but with less strain on the joints.

Maintaining Muscle Mass: Maintaining muscle strength and balance is crucial for staying active and independent as we age. WBV comes to the rescue by offering a fun and effective way to tone those muscles and improve stability. My famous line in my studio was "Use them or lose them".

Studies have shown that WBV can enhance muscle strength and improve balance. Research from Medicine & Science in Sports & Exercise revealed that WBV training significantly improved muscle performance in older adults. The vibrations cause your muscles to contract rapidly, much like they would during conventional resistance training.

Strengthening the Pelvic Floor: Let's be honest, nobody gives you a heads up about this one. Pelvic floor health is increasingly important as we age and affects both men and women. Pelvic floor issues can present itself in many different ways, such as urinary incontinence or pelvic organ prolapse. WBV is particularly beneficial in this area. There are not enough hours in the day to do the number of kegels you would need to get the results of the involuntary muscle contractions that occur while on Power Plate.

In fact, research from the Journal of Family & Reproductive Health concluded that whole-body vibration is an effective way to strengthen pelvic floor muscles. This study focused on the elderly population who often suffer from urinary incontinence. Whole-body vibration training was presented as an intervention to improve pelvic floor muscle strength. The whole-body vibration training group did their 4-week protocol on Power Plate. It was determined that whole-body vibration training may be an effective approach in managing urinary incontinence.

Let It Flow - Boosting Circulation and Enhancing Detoxification

Who doesn't want better circulation and a more efficient lymphatic system? As we age, circulation can become sluggish, leading to various health issues. WBV can give your blood flow and lymphatic drainage the boost they need.

In my wellness studio, clients experienced a 30-minute routine which regularly included about three minutes of stretching to improve flexibility and prepare the muscles for about 18 minutes of work and would always end with massage. Everyone loved the massage. It feels great but the benefits outweigh the fabulous feeling. There were two studies performed at Loma Linda University and published in the Medical Science Monitor.

Increasing Circulation: This study concludes that five minutes of massage on Power Plate at either 30 Hz or 50 Hz significantly increases the skin blood flow and thus circulation in the arms. Performing massage on the 50 Hz setting on Power Plate has additional benefits by increasing the blood flow more rapidly and retaining the level during the recovery period, making the effects longer lasting.

Clinical Applications: Circulation (blood flow) is essential to the human body. Increasing the blood flow to the skin and the tissue beneath it can improve the condition of the skin and firm up skin tone thus helping to reduce the appearance of cellulite. Better circulation is also crucial for healing injured muscles, improving oxygen supply and helping to get rid of waste products, like lactic acid, from the muscles. So, by increasing circulation, massage on a Power Plate can:

- help to improve skin tone.

- reduce the appearance of cellulite.

- encourage muscle recovery after injury.

- help speed recovery after exercise.

Improving Lymphatic Drainage: The gentle vibrations from Power Plate stimulate the lymphatic system, aiding in detoxification and reducing fluid retention. A healthy lymph system is going to remove toxins and waste from the body, boost the immune system and reduce swelling and inflammation. Proper functioning Lymphatic System will contribute to overall better health, increased energy levels and improved recovery from injuries or surgery.

Three months after opening my studio I was diagnosed with a late-stage, rare form of breast cancer. I can tell you first-hand that Power Plate was instrumental in my preparation for surgery and most importantly, my recovery. I had a bilateral double mastectomy with most of my lymph nodes removed from under my left armpit on a Friday in June 2013. The following Monday I was training a light load of clients. I wasn't able to workout right away but I was massaging on vibration every day. One of my greatest risks from that surgery was developing Lymphedema. I celebrated 11 years cancer-free this year and have never had an issue with swelling in my chest or left arm.

Mental Acuity: As we hit our fabulous fifties we should also turn our awareness to brain health. Whole body vibration plays a key role in maintaining or improving mental sharpness. This occurs primarily for two reasons. First, the harmonic vibrations stimulate a neuromuscular response in the body. The brain knows you are on an unstable environment and creates new neural pathways to communicate and trigger the involuntary muscle contractions to stabilize you.

Secondly, is the increase in blood flow to the brain. Restricted blood flow to the brain can lead to serious health issues. When the brain doesn't get enough blood, you may feel dizziness, headaches, confusion, or memory problems. Over time this reduced blood flow may contribute to the development of conditions such as stroke, vascular dementia, and other cognitive impairments.

Research published in the Japanese Society of Nuclear Medicine provides the best evidence and explanation yet of how Power Plate helps keep your brain sharp. Through brain imaging technology, researchers were able to see an increase of blood flow to the frontal region of the brain in people using WBV delivered by Power Plate.

Menopause & Metabolism:

Menopause: Let's be real-this can be a rollercoaster ride that you did not get in line for. Women have different needs when it comes to their wellness and as women get older, they are faced with changing hormone levels due to perimenopause and menopause and other common issues like lower back pain, weakened core, and poor posture.

Menopause induces significant physiological and emotional changes in a woman's body, including hormonal shifts, reduced bone density, muscle mass loss, increased fat accumulation, anxiety, and even depression. These changes can lead to symptoms such as hot flashes, mood swings, decreased metabolism, and weight gain.

As women age, their bodies start playing a mischievous game: piling on extra fat, letting muscle slip away, and moving fat to places it never dared go before. Fortunately, studies published in Maturitas and the Journal of Bone and Mineral Research have shown that WBV, specifically Power Plate training, increases lean tissue, reduces your body fat percentage, improves bone mineral density, increases strength, and improves posture in postmenopausal women.

Resting Metabolic Rate:

Understanding your metabolism or resting metabolic rate is the first step to increasing it. As we age, particularly after the age of 50, our metabolic rate typically decreases. This decline is often associated with several factors, including a reduction in muscle mass, hormonal changes such as decreased estrogen levels (menopause), and a generally more sedentary lifestyle. The basal or resting metabolic rate (BMR), which represents the number of calories the body needs at rest to maintain vital bodily functions, diminishes with age. This decrease in BMR can lead to weight gain if calorie intake is not adjusted accordingly, and it can contribute to a higher risk of metabolic disorders such as type 2 diabetes and cardiovascular disease. As a personal trainer who has helped thousands of clients, I encourage you to know your numbers, especially your BMR. I have found that most women aren't actually taking in enough calories. And when this happens, you actually will gain weight.

Additionally, the decline in muscle mass (sarcopenia) not only lowers metabolism but also impacts strength, balance, and overall physical functionality, making everyday activities more challenging and increasing the risk of falls and fractures.

Here's the cool thing. Whole body vibration training is fast, easy, and creates an immediate metabolic benefit. Just by standing on say, a Power Plate, you stimulate the muscle, and you open up the cells to absorb insulin. When cells are able to use more sugar for energy, you almost instantly solve metabolic problems. Sugar gets used as energy instead of being stored as fat.

Whether you are standing, sitting, or performing exercises on a platform that vibrates at specific frequencies, you stimulate muscle contractions and improve muscle strength and tone. This type of exercise has been shown to enhance metabolic rate by increasing muscle mass and improving muscle function. The vibrations also stimulate blood flow and circulation, which can improve nutrient delivery and waste removal at the cellular level, further supporting metabolic health.

Researchers in Japan have studied and shown that WBV training has been found to have a positive impact on hormone regulation, potentially mitigating some of the adverse effects of menopause, such as reduced estrogen levels. By enhancing muscle mass and improving metabolic efficiency, WBV can help manage weight, reduce the risk of metabolic syndrome, and improve overall physical fitness. Another study published in the European Journal of Applied Physiology evaluated the effects of WBV on body composition and metabolic health. This study demonstrated that WBV could improve body composition by increasing lean mass and reducing fat mass, thereby positively affecting metabolic health.

Balancing Hormones, Balancing Life:

Feel Good Hormones: That just feels good knowing we have "feel good" hormones. I think literally everyday in my wellness studio someone would say to me, "I just feel good when I leave here." Although I would try to explain the science behind why they felt good, it really didn't matter. They were achieving results they had never experienced before.

The truth is the gentle, harmonic vibrations from the Plate boost serotonin and decrease stress hormones like cortisol. High levels of stress hormones encourage fat storage around the abdomen.

Not only does WBV training reduce cortisol but it has been scientifically shown in two different studies to reduce visceral fat. Visceral fat is the bad belly fat. Staying in an optimal range for visceral fat will not only look better on your body but will feel better.

Growth Hormone: Human growth hormone (HGH) is like a special helper in our bodies that helps us grow and stay healthy. It is made by a small part of our brain called the pituitary gland. HGH helps kids grow taller and helps everyone build strong muscles and bones. It also helps our bodies heal when we get hurt and keeps our muscles and fat balanced.

As we get older, our bodies make less HGH. Usually, this starts happening after we turn 30, and the amount keeps getting smaller as we age. When we have less HGH, our muscles might get weaker, our bones can become thinner, and it can be easier to gain weight. This is one reason why people get wrinkles and lose some of their strength as they get older. So, HGH is very important for keeping our bodies strong and healthy throughout our lives.

It is well established that Whole Body Vibration can increase levels of Natural Growth Hormone (GH) in the body by a measurable and meaningful level. Between 400% and 2600% in a range of different studies. It is also well established that once GH levels increase like this, collagen production inside the body goes up. Also, to a measurable and meaningful degree. In a study published in the Journal of Physiology, researchers measured different types of tissue in the body and found that increased levels of GH led to increased levels of Type 1 Collagen and Type 3 Collagen in tendons and skeletal muscle. A journal article in Endocrine Reviews showed increased levels of Collagen in the skin after an increase in GH. What I find interesting is that Type 3 collagen is considered the softer "youth" collagen. We have Type 3 when we are young, and as we get older, the firmer Type 1 makes up 80% of our collagen.

For those of you who have been around the skincare discussion, you know that increases in Type 3 collagen leads to increased skin elasticity, hydration, and firmness. When you use a Power Plate, you are going to increase levels of Growth Hormone in your body naturally. By the way, other forms of intense exercise can also increase GH levels. This is going to lead to some level of increased collagen production in your entire body. Everyone will be different in terms of the exact effects. More collagen in your joints, tendons, and connective tissue is going to keep your body working more comfortably. More collagen in your skin is also a great motivator to start training on Whole Body Vibration. You'll feel good immediately. This is particularly beneficial as HGH plays a crucial role in muscle growth, fat metabolism, and overall physical rejuvenation, which can help older adults maintain muscle mass, reduce body fat, and improve overall metabolic health.

Life is a Balancing Act:

There you have it – the buzz-worthy benefits of whole-body vibration for women of any age. By now, you should be convinced that WBV is more than just a trendy gadget. It's a scientifically backed, fun, and effective way to enhance your health and well-being. Whether you're looking to strengthen your bones, boost your muscle power, improve circulation, or balance those hormones, WBV has got you covered.

As we hit the fabulous decade of our fifties and beyond, we may no longer be juggling kids, spouses, and careers but rather we have to begin balancing our health and well-being. By understanding the physiological changes in our bodies, we can plan the counterattack and naturally improve our biological age. Whole Body Vibration might just be a solution for you.

So why not shake things up and give it a try? Your body will thank you, and you might just find yourself buzzing with energy and vitality. Remember, the journey to lifelong health and happiness is all about finding enjoyable and sustainable ways to stay active. And with WBV, you're just a vibration away from a healthier, happier you. Cheers to shaking it off and embracing a vibrant life!

"I think Power Plate is the fountain of youth."

~Stevie Nicks, American singer-songwriter

About Lisa Dimond

Lisa Dimond is most proud and inspired daily by her two daughters, Veronica and Olivia. Lisa founded and owned BVibrant - A Powerful Wellness Studio in Naples, FL. She is a Certified Power Plate Master Trainer. Although Lisa sold her studio in 2020, she continues to provide cutting-edge technology in the field of health and wellness. She is the co-author of Shine Beyond Cancer. Lisa owns VibrantCEO, a SaaS company that provides marketing solutions to other health and wellness entrepreneurs. For more information on Power Plate or other biohacking devices, please visit https://shinebeyond50.com

Chapter Thirteen

The Tree of Life is Within: Ho'oponopono is the Miracle-Grow

by Caroline Harper

"Yesterday I was clever, so I wanted to change the world. Today I am wise, so I am changing myself."

- Rumi

Just before my 49th Birthday I went to the gynecologist. I had been feeling so tired. Is it my hormones drying up? Vitamin D deficiency? Burnout from 22 years of going in 5th gear as a mom and professional?

"I know you're not due for a pap, but let's just take a little look," she says.

Even after 30 years, I'm still reluctant to get undressed and spread my legs for this particular reason. A cold prying speculum to the vagina always feels like a big look.

She gets in there before poking her head back up. "Well, I can tell you're not in menopause yet because your vagina isn't thinning, and your labia aren't flattening."

"I'm sorry! What's going to happen to my vagina?!"

"The lining thins. It makes it less padded and able to stretch. Sex may become painful."

"Inevitably?"

"Pretty much."

Well, chalk this impression of my shrinking pink lady up to another no one ever told me about menopause moment!

I'm sourly chewing on humble pie, remembering that proud feeling of my youth when I genuinely didn't think even dryness would ever happen to me; just a pity for some "older lady."

I was sure even when I was older, I'd be all lively and horny still like Blanche on The Golden Girls.

On the drive home, the devils on my shoulder with her nagging fears, "So your vagina's going to physically become an unwelcome sign. How's that for a curveball when you're just enjoying the best sex of your life? I hope someone interviews Cardi B and Megan Thee Stallion when they're in their 50s and asks them, 'How do you feel, now that your WAPs aren't so wet?'"

Then I heard from my angel. "Maybe you're drying up is another opportunity to stop looking for fulfillment from things outside yourself and go within for it."

She's soft-spoken but saucy and a little impatient with me. I get it, and I can think of why my angel would be nudging me to go within. She is reminding me of an equation that solves any problem, and life sure had felt problematic recently.

Unlike just a couple years before when we were falling in love, my domestic partner and I were experiencing conflict. Justice had come to me as the answer to a prayer, and became the reward I felt I deserved.

As 2020 began, my oldest daughter received her acceptance to the University of Texas and my youngest turned 16. I had been a single mom for 7 years. Our small town had no dating scene. I'd been using the apps with what felt like a lot of time invested and limited ROI.

Tired of driving long distances to meet strangers I'd only seen pictures of, I prayed a heartfelt wish to meet someone who knew me when I was young. Within 24 hours, like a wave of a fairy godmother's wand, Justice was in my "Liked You" folder.

Justice. Haven't heard that name since... and it looks like him. Oh, Godmother. You are good. I couldn't think who it would be, and you give me Justice?! Glorious.

Before I could put the phone down, he messaged me. After I confirmed it was him, he confessed, "I had a crush on you back then."

We were organizers for an environmental PAC when I was fresh out of UT in the late 90s. I remembered thinking he's the best thing I've ever seen, which hadn't happened before or since.

Little did I know how rare it was! I was young and dumb, and he was as remote as a rock star. Who knows what would have happened if I'd believed I could have the man I wanted, or he'd believed he should follow his instincts. We missed that window.

He loomed large enough in my imagination for a couple of years that when I was pregnant the first time, I suggested his name if we had a boy. My former husband rejected it, and I eventually forgot about him.

I remembered that evening though when he got out of his truck. He came toward me out of a wrinkle in time with that unmistakable walk, like a square-shouldered Marshall in the Wild West giving off "everything's gonna be ok now that I'm in town" vibes. I thought, My God, he's still every bit the man he ever was.

Was I cool as he hugged me in the parking lot? I tried to be. I definitely lost whatever cool I had when we walked into the bar, and he said, "You look the same as you did back then."

My clumsy attempt to return his compliment was, "I was gonna name our baby after you!"

He smiled and said, "Calm down. It's our first date." I almost spit my first sip of wine out laughing. The conversation and laughter between us was warm and natural. It felt strangely new and familiar, how smart and sweet and funny he was.

The year that followed was like re-discovering my best friend. We both love nature and spend as much time as we can in it. We wandered all over, getting lost and found. We laughed a lot and cried some, told each other everything we'd been through, and went through some of the hardest things yet together.

For the first time, I was appreciated completely by a man, and it made me feel covered in the glamor of fairy dust. It was as if I was never fully alive to the things I loved in myself until someone else saw and loved them too. I was laughing at myself -the fairy tale skeptic- for feeling like a Disney princess, but I did. My cup overflowing with love, I poured it out on everyone and everything around me.

And then, as it does, the game of life gave me a whole new level of challenge to clear.

A few months before that visit with my gynecologist, Justice and I bought a fixer-upper, combined our families of 3 daughters, and kicked it off with a 3-week trip through Europe. Think of "Parent Trap" in the "Money Pit" on "European Vacation" and you get some idea of the comedy of errors.

While the environmental chaos and power struggle were binding me up in knots, menopause symptoms came on like a train. I'm wrecked from insomnia, mood swings, and fatigue, but still showing up every day for the task of blending two families of teenage daughters (sharing a bathroom! Under construction!)

Especially in a period of strain or challenge, my devil inside still tricks me into thinking some things are just bad with rants like, "You're in bad shape to get your career back on track post-Covid with that sleepless brain like a fishbowl of Dories swimming around. What are you going to do about the decline in the housing market when you fail at making a peaceful home? That cat and litter box in the bedroom isn't helping the house retain its value or charm either, so you better keep up the pressure about that. You see these things are bad, right? Tell people! They'll tell you!"

It's tempting to believe I'm a victim when I feel scared or weak. I can be a victim of menopause, of the economy, of a questionable housekeeping compromise. It's a comfort to think it's not my fault if things aren't going the way I want.

I can't help but notice, though, how dim the results are in my life when I'm in that mindset. The ethereal glamor of fairy dust was turning into something darker as I told and re-told stories of the bad things happening -to my own brain, to my love, to my family and friends. If truth makes us happy and falsehoods make us weak, I must have been way off track. I took the reminder to heart and used the best, most powerful way I know to go within.

It is a meditation practice that came to me like a blessing straight from grace when I was going through divorce ten years earlier. Slogging through the sucking quicksand of an eroded love in a small southern town, my daughters and I had been surviving, but it was a struggle that went long and deep.

One day the Business Manager of my Unity church gave me a ticket to a weekend event in Austin to thank me for my volunteer efforts at the annual fundraiser.

Attract Money Now Live featured several wonderful speakers teaching about manifestation, the second level of consciousness, or "By Me" mindset. In it, I'm using my creative power over circumstances, shaping what I can to create more of what I want.

The results can be immediate and hard to believe. That job? Seriously! That house? No way! I was just dabbling! Just dreaming!

I was excited to learn all the ways to lift the mind up from the victim mindset, but wasn't expecting an elevator that goes through all the levels of consciousness, from victimhood to enlightenment. This gem was from Joe's second talk on his book, "Zero Limits."

It's the story of an ancient Hawaiian healing ritual to resolve conflicts between people and a modern psychiatrist who healed an entire ward of insane asylum patients by doing it on himself.

Doing what?? What could you possibly do to heal a ward of crazy, violent criminals?

Ho'oponopono, Hawaiian for "to right a wrong," is a family conference, mediated by a kahuna, to address grievances. The goal of the meeting is to obtain the pardon of the offended to receive the higher goal, the pardon of the gods. "Forgive us as we forgive others..."

Hawaiians believe these offenses cause illnesses that can't be cured without reconciliation. Healing comes with complete forgiveness of the whole family. Knowing everyone's physical and mental health was at stake, injured parties come together and make complete apologies with the four phrases. "I'm sorry. Please forgive me. Thank you. I love you," are filled in with whatever responsibility each party takes.

What a solid way to make a full apology and resolve a conflict, right? Makes me think it's why Hawaiians are so chill.

In the 20th century, a Hawaiian kahuna woman named Morrnah Simeona began to teach a new version to the world. She called it Self Identification through Ho'oponopono (SITH). The idea was for individuals to use it on themselves to resolve conflicts.

Kahuna Simeona taught to connect to the gods and the other party in meditation, bringing the wrong to the Divine to be righted and saying the phrases to themselves.

The book is called "Zero Limits" because Morrnah's student, Dr. Ihaleakala Hew Len, said there are none from this place of connection to The Great I AM. He walked the talk with a legendary SITH miracle: taking responsibility for the mental illnesses of a whole ward of criminally insane at the State Hospital in the 1980s.

Dr. Hew Len came to the office every day with a peaceful disposition, but he never met the patients in person. He reviewed their files and said the four phrases to himself, reflecting on their connection to him.

Believing everything in his external environment reflects his internal climate; he worked on forgiving and healing himself. As he "cleared," the patients began to improve. In time, the violent ward became a peaceful environment. Several of the inmates were even successfully rehabilitated into society.

When asked what caused the change, his answer was, "I was simply healing the part of me that created them." He was working on them on that highest "As Me" Level!

Well, that's all good for Dr. Hew Len, who no one is blaming for the mental illness of the asylum patients. Taking responsibility can be a hard thing to do when you feel blamed or wronged. I learned through Ho'oponopono that even if I don't feel responsible for something, I can still take responsibility for it and bring it to the Divine to heal it.

Coming home from the event, I was having a lot of hard feelings in the process of my divorce. My life felt like a ward of criminally insane patients.

I prayed the four phrases because they were simple. I did not feel responsible. I didn't feel the words, but I said them anyway. Like Dr. Hew Len, I focused on the "file" of the "crazy" person and said the four phrases to myself.

I'm sorry. (I don't know what the trolley bucket I ever did to have to fight this hard for less than what the law says is fair.)

133

Please forgive me (for whatever made the father of my children feel wronged to have to support my household after supporting him through the education and business building that afford him his lifestyle.)

Thank you (in advance for working the miracle of your love on a heart that seems turned to stone.)

I love you. (Not him. You God. But you love him, so work your magic.)

Despite my obvious failure to be fully present with the Holy Spirit of unconditional love and forgiveness, the quicksand loosened up. Every time I did SITH, we moved forward a little.

It's the most simple, powerful thing I know to connect with the Great I Am, so powerful you don't even need an open heart. Ho'oponopono opens your heart, wherever it is.

If you've seen Dr. Emoto's work on how water molecules arrange themselves in response to our words and thoughts, you know the base matter of life on earth responds directly to our thoughts and words. "love" and "gratitude" change them into crystalline snowflakes of ordered beauty. "hate" and "evil" become jagged shards of shadowed chaos. If not, please google him to see this concrete proof that when we change the way we look at things, the things we look at change.

Our bodies are also 70% water! The implications of the physiological beauty and order created within us when we evoke the four most positive human emotions are enormous! No wonder the quicksand loosens up—and not just the mental, but the physical, too! The Hawaiian belief in the healing effects of forgiveness on the body doesn't seem so far-fetched.

Western medicine is just catching up to this ancient wisdom of how emotional trauma trapped in the body creates pain and disease.

Even if I use SITH like I did in the divorce -not in deep relationship with The Great I AM, truly repenting, atoning, loving, or feeling grateful, knowing all is for my good- it still works!

Taking responsibility means assuming my God-given power to direct my life. It's the trapeze from the "To Me" to the "By Me" platform, where responsibility comes with great privilege. The first is that I am limited only by my imagination.

I needed to swing myself right back up there from that place where the inner enemy of my joy was attacking my current love life. Differences in how we parent from what food is allowed to where wet towels go had been a regular source of friction.

That morning before I'd left for the Doctor, Justice and I had argued. After treating his daughter to takeout breakfast for the second day in a row, I was telling him how he should limit his spending with helpful tips like, "It's bad to not follow a budget." You can imagine how receptive he was.

On my way home from the Doctor, I saw myself as if from above, wadded up in a pile of frustration that morning. I realized any time I ended up that way, I was focused on getting what I needed outside myself. That feeling of being all balled up and powerless, my love alienated from me is definitely not what I wanted.

Stepping up out of victimhood and meditating with the 4 phrases, I rejected the fear that something bad was happening. If what's happening to me is for my good, then this is an opportunity for growth, to learn, heal, or stretch something.

If I look for the good in what's happening to me, it's always there. The wellness issues of perimenopause could be daunting or an invitation for deep self-care as I enter a new phase of womanhood. An irritation about someone else's over-spending could be an invitation to notice a lack in my own financial responsibility.

Committing to reserve judgment and go within to work when I feel irritated made me happy, so I must have been on to something.

There's no way I would ever let anything shake being on the right path, right? Our love and the peace of our new home were at stake!

That very afternoon, in a fit of bliss, I took it upon myself to sweep and mop the house, do the laundry, cook the family dinner, and clean the kitchen. My back hurt a bit at the end of the day, but I got into bed feeling selfless and satisfied.

In the morning, Justice and I woke up to a text that his daughter wanted to take a shower, and my daughter had left a Band-Aid in the bathtub.

"Can you take care of this?" he asked me.

"Are you serious? Do I look like the Band-Aid maid to you? I can't believe you would ask me that." In my mind, I was being sucked back into the soul-draining vortex of picking up after a whole family. It didn't feel good.

"It's not my Band-Aid," he defended, blissfully unaware I'm going over an edge he didn't push me to.

"It's not mine either! I guess you think I'm here to clean up after everyone, just to cook and clean and do your bidding! That's what you treat me like!" I left for a walk before saying anything else.

The story was starting to blow up in my head. I can't even believe with all I do around here that I'm rung up to collect some petty trifle, like a servant. This is a bad situation. It's when I heard the words "bad situation," I became aware I was doing it again

I stopped trying to clean the mess on the screen I'm projecting and turned to the projector with repentance, forgiveness, gratitude, love. The four phrases are a wonderful pattern interrupt to fearful thoughts whenever they come up.

As I say them a calm always comes over me. The more time I spend in that second level of consciousness, the more I bump up against the third. Higher truth finds its way in that space. No one asked you to do all that housekeeping yesterday, or anything but to "take care of" a Band-Aid being in the tub -and they are gross after all! Could it be a sign of something needing healing?

I saw that I had projected this lowly housekeeper persona, and realized there was work to do on a past me who did too much for too long without speaking up for the support she needed. I said the four phrases, forgiving and giving myself the love I needed. As I did, it was easier to think of ways to handle the current need differently.

Back home, I grabbed a five-dollar bill, pen, and paper and went up to the bathroom. Exchanging the Band-Aid for the bill, I left a note that said, "I'll pay up this time, but all future rewards depend on the goods being left in the trash can. - The Band-Aid Fairy."

I sent a text to my daughter, "There's something for you in the bathroom!"

She came in to me videoing her finding the money and note. After reading it, she pockets the money and hugs me "Sweet! Another revenue stream!"

"Hopefully there won't be too much money to be made there."

She laughed and shrugged, "I can be clumsy."

"You don't really want someone else to have to throw away your used bandage, do you?"

"No, mom. I'm sorry. It won't happen again."

I went downstairs and showed the video to Justice. He laughed at the goofy face she made stashing the bill and said "I hope she doesn't think bigger Band-Aids mean more money." His playful smile confirmed I'd done more to build a team than arguing with him about who does more cleaning.

The only thing that ever takes me out of being joyful and carefree in life is when I judge something as bad. Believing that life is good and that something bad is happening are like sneezing and keeping my eyes open. I can't do them at the same time.

It is the morale in the Adam and Eve parable.

In the Paradise God made, there are two trees. One is blessed and the other forbidden. There's the Tree of Life. As long as we eat its fruit, we are happy with all our needs provided for in shameless love, abundance, and connection to God.

In the other corner, there's the Tree of Knowledge of Good and Evil. Its fruit makes us think we are like gods, knowing what's good and bad. Judgment leads to condemnation, blame and shame that pave the road to suffering, our hearts and ears closed to God.

The Garden is still there. The key to those higher states of consciousness, that Heaven at hand, is to enjoy everything but judgment. That third level of Surrender Consciousness takes faith in the goodness of God, even in the face of everything. That's the fruit of life.

I'm clear the other fruit is bitter, so I'm doing my best to stick to this diet. Temptation to judge comes back up on the regular, though. The separate self returns to submerge the Higher Self with the false beliefs and stories it fears. "Look at all the danger out there!" is her relentless unwelcome focus.

Taking control got me out of victimhood, but to get to cooperate with the Divine, I have to let it go. Relying on my intuition, I let love and healing "Through Me." Unlike on the second level where I am limited by my imagination, the possibilities here are beyond the imagination because an all-knowing all-powerful limitlessly creative force is working through me. All it takes is believing everything that happens to me is for my good.

Anything that takes me out of that is pointing me back to the work inside me, cleaning up condemnation, lack of self-love, and unforgiven things, remembering the truth of who I AM. Maybe one day I'll run out of reasons to go within, but for now, every time I feel "triggered," there's an inside job to do.

Had I let separate self-drive in the Band-Aid incident, I'd have done all the things First Corinthians says love is not, starting with self-seeking and culminating in keeping a record of wrongs. If the past is any indication, that would put me on Rocky Road heading toward Alien Nation.

I do my best to subdue her and keep her from driving, even though she sounds like she knows what's ahead. If I look back on all the times I believed something bad was happening that were for my good -jobs I left, relationships that ended- I can think of a few.

Everything coming at me is just life with its lessons for me. I affirm it's all good, go back to the whiteboard, and pray the four phrases of Ho'oponopono. When I go within, I'm doing everything in my power and inspiring others I might want to fix or change to do the same. Best of all, I actually do change them. Through my connection to them and the Divine, I can direct my love right to their water molecules.

Ho'oponopono is rooted in the belief that we are all one energy. It is the highest form of self-love and selfless love in one to heal a rift in that energy with forgiveness.

The more I'm mindful that I am one with everyone and everything, the easier it is to say, "Please forgive me." It's become my daily prayer. A drop of cosmic plasma, I expand my awareness to the vast ocean, recognizing this is not a thing outside me, but myself. "Thank you."

The nature of this ocean of I AM is a benevolent force of love, abundance, beauty, creation, and eternal life. I can access this direct relationship at any time. Living the truth that "Everything in the Cosmos great and small lives in the Self - the source of life," I am unfuckwithable. "I love you."

The solution is always, I AM the way and the light. Don't think you have to wait until you're drying up to go within and lift your consciousness. It's always the right time to release struggle and choose life.

It feels and looks better, keeping faith that everything is constructed for my good. Anything that doesn't feel like it gets to come with me to get cleaned up by my love.

That feels like a solid way to head into my 50 and Fabulous Era. I'm giving all my fucks to me. Not the literal ones. Just the figurative.

About Caroline Harper

Caroline Harper is a writer and teacher, a seeker of truth, and a champion of mercy. A Licensed Minister and Certified Advanced Ho'oponopono Practitioner, she teaches connection to power and purpose. Through public events, workshops, private sessions, and retreats, she helps people create lives they love with their God-given gifts. Connect on IG @YouAreTheFirebird

Chapter Fourteen

Live Your Brilliance! 5 Steps to Creating Your Best Life After 50

By Susan J. Rosenthal

Living your brilliance is your birthright! You are meant to shine. You were not created to lead a life of quiet desperation or boredom. You deserve happiness, freedom, peace, and fulfillment. All of this was yours the moment you took your very first breath.

BUT… how easy it is to succumb to family pressure, relationship pressure, or societal expectations and lose yourself to the daily grind. As women, we are very vulnerable to the trap of ignoring our authentic selves as we attempt to fulfill roles and obligations not all of our own making. And, wow, are we persistent at our self-denial! Doing for ourselves gets pushed to the bottom of the priority list (or possibly gets bumped off the list altogether).

At 50 and beyond, women already have decades of selfless behavior (and plenty of social reinforcement for it) behind them. The patterns of self-denial and going above and beyond for others can often feel like they are cased in concrete and can never be broken.

Women are so good at helping others shine brilliantly. We strive to be perfect partners, wives, mothers, sisters, grandmothers, friends, and co-workers. In our 50s and beyond, we are generous caregivers and babysitters. Women with careers also find themselves giving their all to everyone except themselves. It can be a vicious cycle. The more women give, the less we have to give to ourselves. Our authentic selves seem to fade away into a distant memory.

Are you trapped forever on the treadmill? No! Our authentic essence didn't evaporate; it just got boxed up somewhere inside. How do we reclaim that wonderful, talented woman we locked in the basement for the sake of others? Can we, at long last, make ourselves priorities in our own lives?

YES, WE CAN! So, let's get to it!

When is the right time to put yourself at the forefront of your life and focus on YOU? I have discussed this question countless times with clients, colleagues, and friends. In juggling the elements of a full life, women frequently, consciously or unconsciously, put the priorities, needs, and expectations of others ahead of their own. The requirements of raising a family, building a career, paying bills, managing the house, caregiving parents, nurturing friendships, and numerous other obligations can lead women to place their own interests and self-care on hold.

Turning 50 was a wake-up call for me. Just ten days after my birthday, while working out of town, a sudden illness caused me to lose the sight in one of my eyes. My doctor issued an ultimatum: change my lifestyle and habits or potentially face a life-changing, long-term health condition. My options sounded limited and dire.

Here was the irony: I was successful and had big plans for the future. I was living the life of achievement that I had craved for so many years. But that success was slowly killing me physically and spiritually. I had much of what I wanted …only to feel disconnected from the true and best version of myself. This was no longer a sustainable vision of life for me. I felt lost and confused. Okay, the old vision was no longer working… but how do I find a new one?

The silver lining was this became a catalyst for personal growth and a healthier lifestyle. You could say that losing my physical vision was a pathway to finding a new and vibrant vision for my own life and for others. I not only became an advocate for my own healing but surveyed many aspects of my life – across mind, body, emotions and spirit. Happily, my eyesight returned in just over a year with minimal medical intervention. Below, I will share several key elements that guided my growth and healing and led to a more harmonious, balanced, and joyful second half of life.

To start, let's glance back several decades.

Growing up, I was raised with Midwestern values. I was taught that focus and hard work would enable me to attract the opportunities to fulfill my goals and dreams. On the one hand, it seemed that I was living the life of an independent and empowered woman. I went to college and then earned a master's degree in business. I worked at the senior management level within several large and successful corporations. With dedication and perseverance, I enjoyed career success beyond anything my mother and grandmothers could have imagined for themselves.

However, external and social influences were less open-minded and promising. Popular media advised women to be attractive and valuable through serving others, whether at home, work or in society. News, ads, and television shows encouraged women to focus on their desirability and self-improvement over self-worth and success. We were taught to mold ourselves to fit in and be grateful for what we receive, which included less pay and fewer opportunities than our male peers.

What had seemed like a wonderful new world of opportunities for women started feeling like a trap. We had to work harder than men. We had to be perfect in what we said and did. We had to dodge unwanted advances from men in power. The promise of equal opportunity was, at best, only half fulfilled.

The successes in my 30s, 40s, and 50s came with working excruciatingly long hours and leading a hectic, full life. Focused on being productive more than happy, I devoted limited time outside of family and work to rest and play. Being honest, the overfull life treadmill left me anxious, tired, depressed, and burned out before reaching 50. I knew I couldn't continue on this path and thrive. How had I drifted so far from my passions and happiness? It became imperative to explore myself inside, gain a deeper understanding, and return to focusing on me.

This process of re-discovery and renewal was challenging work, but it was joyful work. With each new insight about the real me, I felt that much more fulfilled, confident and happy.

Back to the initial question: When is the right time to put yourself at the forefront of your own life and live your own brilliance? Now, of course!

Women are generally taught that 50 is the end of our useful, productive life. There is nothing important for us to do after 50 but accept our diminished relevance and find activities to keep us occupied. Life does not have to be this way! It should not be this way! We can embrace this second stage of our life as the gift that it is. We are not winding down. With our hard-earned wisdom and experiences, plus our talents and dreams, we are just getting warmed up!

"But wait," you might say. "Won't it take years, maybe decades, to unwind a past full of stress and self-denial?"

Happily, the answer is a resounding "NO!" You can start right here, right now! The path back to your true self and authentic brilliance follows five steps. This is a path of joyful discovery, not pain and drudgery. So, if you're ready to connect to your authentic self, take some deep cleansing breaths and get ready to be amazed at the incredible woman you are about to rediscover!

5 STEPS TO LIVE YOUR BRILLIANCE

STEP 1: REDISCOVER

Jeanene, a 51-year-old mother of two and manager at a technology security firm, came to me weighed down with frustration and discontent. She enjoyed her work challenges and was recently awarded a promotion, but work was taking too much time away from her family and herself. Beyond that, Jeanene's enthusiasm and ambition had waned. She felt she was not fulfilling her purpose, though she was not clear on what it was. In the months that we worked together, Jeanene reclaimed herself and learned what brings her joy and makes her unique. She rediscovered her purpose and took steps to actively incorporate it into her daily life.

When you feel out of harmony or alignment with yourself and your inner essence or purpose, it is easy to disconnect from yourself. You may find yourself saying "one day I will…"., "if only I could…", "I wish …", or even descending into a negative mindset. These thoughts take you out of the present moment and can distract you from creating your best life.

Age 50 and beyond is an ideal time to look inside and rediscover what defines you and lies at the core of your essence. It is a time to reclaim you as you reach for what makes your heart sing, enlivens your dreams, and makes you shine.

Reclaiming your authentic essence is an intentional process of choosing to focus on you - knowing who you are and what you want in your present and future life. This is done more easily by studying yourself at the levels of mind, body, emotions, mind, heart, and spirit. Allow yourself to embrace joyfully your passions and drives. Also, face up to the false beliefs about yourself, ingrained routines, and external pressures that inhibit you, frustrate you, and block your inner path to your authentic self.

To reclaim yourself means that you intentionally put yourself at the center of your life. You get to redesign your life to align with who and where you are right now, and who you want to be. How wonderful is that? These amazing insights provide a strong foundation to refine or redesign your extraordinary path toward living your own brilliance and joy. Start by reclaiming who you truly are!

STEP 2: HEAL

As a divorced 62-year-old woman, Kristina was filled with regret, anger, and grief. She was stuck in an endless loop of self-evaluation and rethinking past decisions. Kristina felt boxed in by self-imposed judgments and limitations set by employers, family, relationships, and finances. She could not get out of her own way to pursue new thoughts, dreams, and opportunities. In developing a new path for her happiness and healing, Kristina learned to manage her thoughts and emotions and to, most importantly, accept and love herself.

While experiencing circumstances outside of your control and comfort zone, it is easy to let old thoughts, feelings and habits sabotage your wholeness and happiness. You may be unaware of internal and external beliefs, criticism and doubts that affect you all day every day. Many of these were seeded as you grew up, now ready to be triggered at any moment.

The ability to undergo change, focus on passion, and pursue a life you desire is greatly influenced by your relationship with yourself. It may be time to heal your past or present thoughts and emotions, let go of resistances and self-doubt, and free yourself to embrace new directions.

STEP 3: REJUVENATE

Aarya had an autoimmune condition, low energy, and was feeling physically depleted at 54 years old. She talked about having lost her excitement and sense of adventure in life. Aarya played an active role in her children's lives, providing support and babysitting whenever they needed. At the same time, she gave care to her mother undergoing cancer treatment. Working together, Aarya created a plan for her physical and emotional rejuvenation, including Pilates, dance classes, and planning more social engagements. These restored her energy, reignited her sense of fun, and re-motivated her to pursue a passion project she had dreamed about since childhood.

After 50 is a great time to assess your energy level, motivation, and overall wellbeing to discern if you are in need of renewal or rejuvenation. Continually giving to others while not replenishing yourself can often lead to depletion, irritability, burn out or illness.

By the time we reach our 50s and beyond, we have experienced numerous life changes and events. Your ongoing habits, thoughts, emotions and self-image may no longer align with who you currently are. Having processes to update these so they reflect your own truth can be illuminating, energy building and joyful.

Self-care is also important for your long-term health and sustainability. Making time to boost your physical and mental health can be the support you need to pursue your dreams and take bold actions. Scheduling time for relaxation, massages, or other forms of self-pampering and play is an act of self-love and a proactive approach to keeping you in alignment with yourself. Don't wait until you are depressed, frustrated, or depleted. A continual habit of renewal and replenishment will improve your life, fuel your dreams, and let your light shine bright.

STEP 4: REFOCUS

Work had become unbearable for Hallie, a 57-year-old healthcare professional. She lost her passion for her work due to the restrictive governmental and legal requirements. In addition, her company was a nightmare with politics, budget reductions, and in-fighting. Hallie was ready for a drastic change but lacked clarity on the direction that would make her happy. For several years, she had considered launching her own consulting business. She realized this was the right time to step back and go through a process of refocusing on the dreams, passions and lifestyle which could allow her to thrive.

After 50, many women reach a point where we feel stuck or bored. We may be experiencing excessive levels of stress or frustration. We can feel like we are just treading water or that we have outgrown the appeal we once held. Or we may lack enthusiasm in our relationships, careers, outside interests, or just life in general. We are ready for something different and more fulfilling.

Refocusing is a deep dive process to understand your passions and needs in the here and the now. Your inner wisdom can offer you the clarity and the answers you need. At the same time, you can practice setting boundaries. You can empower yourself by saying "yes" to what you do want in your life and "no" to what no longer serves you.

Honor your own needs and allow yourself to be joyfully selfish. Wait! Isn't it wrong to be selfish? This is not a selfishness of self-absorption or egocentricity, but a vehicle to discover and fulfill your personal desires while embracing the power within you. By allowing yourself to refocus on you, your personal self-worth, happiness, and peace can expand exponentially.

STEP 5: REINVENT

At 63 years old, Maddie felt like joy and time had run out for her when she became a widow. Life plans came to a halt when her husband succumbed to heart disease. Maddie cut her work hours to part-time in order to focus on getting her life on track. She initially set out to fill it with travel, gardening, and spending time with people she loved. Maddie soon realized she wanted more purposeful activities and to rebuild her life around unfulfilled desires. At the same time, she felt she was too established in her ways to create herself anew. Maddie sought help to get out of her own way and open up to new possibilities. Her reinvention was a beautiful process that energized her to want to live another 25 years, making every moment count.

When we hit 50, are we pretty much set in our ways? Will our patterns and beliefs from the past drive us forever? Only if we let them.

You may not realize it, but you have the power to continually clear the past, heal in the present, and reinvent yourself. In fact, reinventing aspects of yourself on an ongoing basis can add to your vitality as you bring your dreams and desires to life.

Giving yourself permission to move in a new direction is an act of self-ownership and self-empowerment. You have the ability to change how you view your reality and experience and, in doing so, influence your possibilities to create yourself anew.

Dreaming big, taking risks, and making new choices are elements of self-mastery. Simply accept what has been true your whole life: you are amazing! Embrace your power and your vitality. Your wisdom and creativity are limitless. Use your gifts, experience, and essence to redesign your own future.

Lastly, you have the power in every minute to make new choices. Once you do, commit to them. YOU are the solution to fulfilling your own needs and desires. Think of yourself as a winner and watch yourself become that awesome woman you choose to be!

REDISCOVER! HEAL! REJUVENATE! REFOCUS! REINVENT!

These are the signposts on the path to realizing your brilliance. I discovered these signposts with a lot of hard work and some trial and error. One step forward was often followed by two steps back. Now, you don't have to feel your way along the path. There is much more to rediscovering yourself and creating your journey to brilliance than can be covered in one chapter. I want to be there for you and provide all the support, guidance, and tools to help you become the person you want to be.

In choosing to put yourself first after 50, you CAN create an extraordinary, fulfilling and happy life. You will share and give to others from a genuine spirit of generosity and joy, not from an imposing sense of over-responsibility. In any moment, you have a chance to awaken, envision and create a life you love.

As they say, it's the journey, not the destination. The joy of self-discovery and reinvention can be a permanently joyful way of living. Every day, you transform into a new version of yourself by means of your experiences and ways of being. Use these five steps to liberate yourself from all that holds you back. Watch with wonder and awe as your authentic and joyful self blossoms. Wielding your amazing power to make intentional choices and take deliberate actions will empower you to live your own brilliance.

Dance! Laugh! Sing! Create! Love! Live with gratitude for your life and the amazing gifts and experiences it brings you. And, if you desire, you will find ways to live and give to the world that do not diminish you, but engage your spirit and fill your heart.

Your life is a big, beautiful adventure at 50 and beyond. Embrace it! Cherish it! Love it!

About Susan J. Rosenthal:

Susan Rosenthal is a global leader at the crossroads of personal development, business and spirituality. She has guided individuals, teams and organizations through growth and transformation as a mentor, coach, business executive and consultant. Susan has an MBA from Northwestern University and is a Certified Life Coach and Certified Business Coach. As a Certified Professional Speaker (CPCS), Susan also speaks at international events and conferences. She was featured in the book, Fearless Women: Visions of a New World, and at the Fearless Women Global Conference. In addition, Susan is co-author of Infinite Footprints: Daily Wisdom to Ignite Your Creative Expression in Walking Your True Path, a practical, guided journey of self-discovery, personal freedom and authentic expression. She is an active board member for multiple organizations that elevate women and girls' economic development, education, health and empowerment worldwide.

Chapter Fifteen

Navigating Aging with Grace, Strength, and Mobility: You Can Only Be Strong in the Range of Motion You Have

by Diane Waye

Have you ever noticed that children take long, fluid strides while walking and running, but many adults take shorter steps, mostly just in front of their bodies?

The demands of 'modern life' often require only small motions but maintaining our full Range of Motion (ROM) with strong, healthy muscles is valuable to the quality of our lives, from our ease of walking to our comfortable joints to our even better sex!

Owning our full ROM helps prevent muscle and joint injuries and empowers us to participate in our chosen activities. Using our muscles enhances our mood, brain power, and overall health. We must move and strengthen our muscles through exercise and play to thrive.

Why Muscles Matter:

Did you know skeletal muscles are considered endocrine organs? Muscles motor every action we make, from reading to walking, yet muscles also produce growth factors, myokines, irisin, and other valuable substances that boost health. They help regulate body temperature and stabilize critical hormones like insulin and cortisol. Muscle activity triggers peptide release, DNA repair, and the production of anti-inflammatory cytokines. Additionally, muscle action stimulates the production of testosterone and other hormones by influencing glandular activity. Regular physical activity even reduces the risk of certain cancers. Muscle health is essential to our well-being, especially as we age.

With all the vital substances they make, it's worth noting that our wonderful muscles rely on a hormone they don't produce, estrogen, for optimal function and repair. To thrive, I supplement my Mediterranean diet with creatine and HRT. If HRT isn't your preference or an option for you, that's all the more reason to double down on exercise and other healthy self-care! You do you.

I recently witnessed a young paraplegic woman's inspirational journey to pull-ups. You can start where you are and lovingly expand your fitness journey for your fabulous future!

Better Brains:

Exercise has neuro-protective qualities for our brain health.

Is this due to infusing our brain tissue with oxygen? BDNF's? Or because people who exercise tend to sleep soundly? (Our brain's cleaning system is considered most active during sleep when flushing out waste products such as those characteristics of Alzheimer's disease.)

"Exercise has Immediate, long-lasting, and protective benefits for your brain," says Dr. Wendy Suzuki, brain plasticity specialist, professor of Neural Science and Psychology, and TED speaker. (As someone with nearly four decades of experience in the fitness profession, I love that Dr. Suzuki earned her fitness certification after her PhD, inspired by studying the effects of exercise!)

Psychological Well-Being:

Did you know you have an epic internal "pharmacy"? We make serotonin, oxytocin, dopamine, endorphins, and melatonin. Engaging in physical activity triggers the release of these chemicals that promote psychological well-being.

Strength training requires focus on the present, which can soothe rumination and anxiety. Cardio calms. Combining mindful movement with intentional breathing is likely to uplift your mood.

I enjoy structured exercise, but I love play too! Play exponentially multiplies many benefits of exercise, especially mood-elevating rewards. Did you know that Play enhances cognitive function? Play helps us learn!

Hula hooping may seem frivolous, yet it is fun, core-centric, and encourages mindfulness, your hoop will drop if your mind wanders. Monkey bars are ideal for lengthening while strengthening, and they promote coordination. Skipping may seem silly, but I double-dare you to stay in a bad mood while skipping! (Plus, skipping is plyometric like jumping; plyometrics significantly increases growth hormone secretion.)

Did you know that EMDR was developed by a psychotherapist who observed improvements in her patients during walks? This lateral eye movement therapy helps take the "charge" off trauma. Walking works. Time outdoors under an open sky nourishes our whole being in many ways!

Better Bones:

Muscles move bones - and they tug on our bones, which helps our bones stay strong! You don't have to pound the pavement or do high-impact aerobics to stimulate bone strength - even non-weight-bearing activities (such as swimming) promote bone density.

And did you know that bones aren't "just" skeletal structures? Our bones are busy building blood, storing minerals, and synthesizing Vitamin D for starters. And they remodel themselves -- bones truly are dynamic organs!

One of my 80-year-old clients saw a 3% increase in her bone density six months from when we restored her mobility. Bone density was a powerfully positive yet "unintended consequence" of our sessions. (Dorie's story is below.)

Heart & Lungs:

Your heart is arguably the most important muscle in your body - it pumps blood out.

Did you know that other muscles assist in bringing it back? So don't resist the urge to tap your toes on long flights! Lifting your forefoot (with your knees bent) is even more specific for stimulating the deep calf to pump blood from your legs back towards your heart. The anatomical name of this strategically located muscle is "Soleus," but its medical nickname is "The Second Heart"! So the next time you're stuck in a seat, activate your leg pump "heart" with a few sets of ten "forefoot lifts" to promote circulation.

Breath is life, but "reduced breathing capacity" is "accepted" as part of aging. Because this is primarily due to losing elasticity in the diaphragm and ribs and not exhaling fully, you have some agency in dodging this statistic! Engage in breathing exercises to fortify your respiratory function and oxygenate your system.

Have you ever noticed how a yawn, sigh, or even a good cry can help you feel better? You can intentionally activate this mechanism with a practice called "The Cyclic Sigh." Our lungs contain 300-500 million tiny air sacs called alveoli, essential to gas exchange. Alveoli sometimes partially collapse, and because they are sticky, they benefit from a blast of air to re-inflate. The "Cyclic Sigh" pops open our alveoli to push air in.

Here's how to do it: Take a double or triple inhale (through your nose if possible), "overfilling" your lungs, followed by a slow and complete exhale through your mouth.

Even a few such breaths improve oxygenation!

The cyclic sigh is an easy antidote for "email apnea" and is proven to reduce stress. Yet it is only one of many breathing exercises you can engage in! Why not try it now?

Posture is also crucial to breathing well.

Immune & Lymphatic System Functioning:

Moving our muscles benefits our immune system by enhancing lymphatic drainage. Lymph channels run parallel to blood vessels, allowing lymph to monitor blood. The lymphatic system helps eliminate toxins, transports cancer cells to collection sites, and removes waste. It also fights infections and maintains fluid balance in the body. Muscle contractions from physical activity stimulate lymph flow, supporting this vital system's functionality to help keep us clean and healthy inside.

Metabolism:

Muscles are a valuable tool for managing weight and fueling energy. Muscle tissue uses more energy (calories) even at rest than non-muscle tissue. While "burning calories" may seem like a luxury problem, maintaining a good metabolism is crucial for preventing or managing type 2 diabetes.

Better Sex:

Energizing our whole body regularly is conducive to enjoying sex. And so is a comfortable ROM! I'm not suggesting gymnastics in bed unless it is genuinely part of your "desire," but you don't want to be limited by discomfort!

A 25-year-old athlete who attended my recent seminar told me later that stretching her inner thighs allowed her to enjoy sex without distraction from tight muscles. Similarly, when I learned the basic "pelvic tilt" exercise at her age, I got to enjoy sex without any low back bother. Plus, mastering the pelvic tilt allows me more precision of angles for targeting pleasure! Having a baseline of good health, including an easy, comfortable ROM, makes sexual enjoyment and exploration easier. Sex after 50 should be about pleasure and nourishing health.

Mastering Kegel exercises is beneficial regardless of interest in sexual activities. Please note that other exercises of the hip region should not be confused with Kegels or pelvic floor exercises, as they foster different benefits. (Even the "pelvic tilt" is not a pelvic floor exercise!) Additionally, it's essential to understand that Kegels, like all exercises, have both a strengthening and relaxation phase. (If you have persistent pelvic floor pain, please consult with your doctor.)

Better Sleep:

How do we get kids to sleep? We encourage activities to tire them out. We never outgrow our need for exercise!

(Exercise enhances sleep; however, if you are newly returning to the wonderful world of exercise, you'll likely sleep best if you do your cardio in the first half of your day.)

Why Range of Motion (ROM) Matters:

You can only be strong in the Range of Motion (ROM) you have. If you strengthen only in a partial range, you will still reap benefits from cultivating your muscles (yay!), but you might compromise your joints, nerves, and future freedom of movement.

In the stride length scenario, it's simply a matter of opening tight muscles on our front sides & getting our backsides engaged. (Literally & figuratively!) We need to maintain or reclaim the follow-through portion of our gait. There are stretching and strengthening exercises to restore proper gait, yet simply walking backward can activate your glutes, priming them for greater follow-through engagement! If you've been neglecting the final third of your stride, you'll still need to be mindful to use your glutes for follow-through when walking frontwards (for a while).

Nerves don't like being squished. When squished temporarily, they shoot "stingers" or tingle. There's nothing "funny" about a "funny bone" zinger - but at least it passes quickly!

Squishing spinal discs can cause lingering collateral damage, such as sciatica (or worse). Most nerves exit the spine, passing spinal discs on their path to parts they innervate. Maintaining proper space and stability for the segments of our spine makes this passage easy for our nerves. Some popular "core" exercises can be stressful to the lumbar spine, but don't worry - there are safe and effective options! Notice sensations you feel, and honor the wisdom of your body.

Full ROM is rarely required daily in most modern lifestyles, so we must train and use it (or lose it)!

Stretching:

Stretching is my known specialty! I use Active Isolated Stretching (AIS) to achieve ROM and follow up with Active Isolated Strengthening. (Both are The Mattes Method.) This ensures that lengthened muscles are also strong and functional.

AIS is based on neurological science such as Nobel Prize-Winning Sherrington's Law of Reciprocal Inhibition, which states that when a muscle contracts, its direct agonist (opposite) relaxes to an equal extent. This prevents muscles from working against each other.

AIS also respects the importance of The Stretch Reflex, which gets triggered when a muscle's tendon senses inappropriate stretching. Most stretch systems override this reflex, yet doctors test for it because of its protective value. The famous rubber mallet knee-tap tests the body's response to sudden stretches.

When clients come to me seeking hands-on assisted stretching, they're often unfamiliar with the Active Isolated Stretching (AIS) technique. It's a joy for me to introduce them to The Mattes Method of AIS and witness their "aha" moment" when they realize how much sense AIS makes, how effective it is, and how good it feels!

The repetition of AIS oxygenates muscles gives them an elastic, springy texture- what Tom Brady calls "pliability." Athletes especially love AIS because it enables them to achieve their full potential. An athlete can only be strong in the ROM she can access!

AIS is easy self-care, too! My YouTube channel started as a collection of single-stretch videos for my clients in their homes.

AIS is an amazing tool with many uses! AIS nourishes muscles and meridians!

Some of my clients had complex challenges that AIS has been able to help with as well.

Hypermobility and Hypomobility:

"Good flexibility" means optimal joint range of motion (ROM) governed by healthy muscles. This is also great for mobility. On the other hand, when I say "bad flexibility," I don't mean a lack of flexibility." I'm referring to "ligament laxity" (loose ligaments) or hypERmobility. Ligament laxity can leave joints unstable and more vulnerable to injuries. The good news is that muscles can be trained to compensate for ligament laxity, literally "taking up the slack" to stabilize the joints in place of the lax ligaments. Muscles to the rescue (again!)

A joint is what we call a place where bones meet. Joints come in a variety of shapes. Shapes govern how they prefer to glide, slide, hinge, and rotate. We must respect how each joint is designed to function and its ideal ROM. Joints thrive with a balance of freedom and structural integrity. Joints need space so the cartilage (on the ends of bones where they meet other bones) can move well. Synovial fluid is lubricated in and for our joints; movement is how we stimulate this lubrication.

It is important to understand the difference between tendons and ligaments. Ligaments' primary purpose is to connect bone to bone and to guide (like soft guard rails) the joint action. Ligaments contribute to proprioception by providing sensory feedback about joint position and movement. Tendons are the tapered ends of muscles that connect to the bones they move. Tendons and their muscles have even more functions related to sensory feedback (through mechanisms such as the stretch reflex). Tendons play a significant role in proprioception, which is" the body's ability to sense its position, motion, stability, and balance.

We want to stretch muscles, not ligaments or nerves. If you have tight muscles and want to improve your joint ROM, your healthy "stretch-ability" can be easily cultivated.

I have a zig-zag spine condition called "idiopathic scoliosis," which runs in my family. My mother experienced debilitating discomfort from her scoliosis, so I've prioritized being proactive to feel good. Hence, my lifelong exploration of movement, stretching, and function!

The connection between scoliosis and hypermobility is recognized medically in Europe more than in my country. However, in my personal and clinical experience, I've found hypermobility to be a significant factor. Although only a tiny percentage of the population has to navigate scoliosis per se, many people have some degree of hypERmobility, such as hypERextension at the knees (sometimes called "locking out"). By learning proper joint alignment and avoiding hyperextension, most people experience greater comfort in their backs, knees, and necks!

Understanding the ideal range of motion for each joint and how it impacts your comfort and the whole structure is empowering. You can then cultivate a healthy level of flexibility, address any excessive ranges with targeted exercises, and consciously make any adjustments necessary for optimal alignment.

Strengthen throughout your optimal ROM for best results:

Building on the cornerstone of strength through ROM, train to mitigate any repetitive movements or suboptimal postures of your work, sports, and hobbies. Don't be shy about training in aesthetics, too! But cover the basics first. Strengthening through ROM is akin to mastering musical scales before improvising in a genre that inspires you.

Pro Tip: Strengthening throughout full ROM tends to sculpt long-looking muscles!

Some of my clients had complex challenges:

Dorie:

While volunteering at the Y, I met a lovely 80-year-old named Dorie, who taught chair yoga there. Watching her walk, I understood why she taught yoga in a chair. So I offered my help. She had a "stuck" hip from a car accident decades earlier. Because her hip was "frozen" in flexion, she kept her opposite knee bent to balance her babies on her hip, so one knee was also "frozen/stuck."

Additionally, her toes were "hammered" due to the pointy-toed high-heels female bank tellers were expected to wear "back in the day." In just a few (long) sessions, we restored function to all her joints, freeing her from pain! Dorie was thrilled to put her newfound mobility to good use by taking long walks with her friends and having adventures. Six months later, she phoned with additional good news -- her bone density had improved by 3%.

Liz:

Liz sought help for her hip, but she also had significant forward curvature in her upper spine (called kyphosis), plus scoliosis, like myself. Towards the beginning of our sessions together, Liz told me she'd never found stretching helpful before, but AIS felt good to her! A few months into our work, she excitedly announced, "I'm no longer looking down at the ground when I walk! How nice to enjoy a view of the horizon "and get taller incrementally week after week at 67!" Sometimes, Liz comes in with a specific goal, such as pain relief from a shoulder injury caused by rowdy children. This prioritized improving her overall shoulder alignment. My approach involves releasing restricted areas, strengthening the opposite muscles, and strengthening what we've freed. I love working with Liz because she's creative, curious, and always inspired to integrate what I teach her! We are both intrigued by the body's marvelous malleability!

Invest in Your Body's Mobility Retirement Fund:

If exercise were a pill, it would be The Best-Seller for sexual pleasure, sleep, mental health, metabolism, the health of your heart, brain, bones, and your quality of life! But the benefits of exercise can't be bought in a bottle.

You can exercise with friends, strangers, or alone. You can work out and play in a facility, at home, or outdoors. You can hire people to guide and coach your exercise, but you can't pay them to do it for you. Muscles are forged through activity.

In the second half of your life, free from pressure to participate in a particular sport, it's your choice how you want to move your body. The world is your gym and playground!

As you cultivate your muscle organs, remember that maintaining strength throughout the optimal range of motion is important to your body's MOBILITY. Don't let your world or your stride length shrink. The classic proverb states, "The best time to plant a tree is 20 years ago, but the second to best time is now". So, from wherever you are, lovingly expand your fitness journey into the fabulous future you deserve.

About Diane Waye

Diane Waye empowers people to achieve greater health through speaking, on-site presentations, AIS professional education seminars, and sessions. (Therapeutic sessions are hands-on or Zoom.)   https://stretchingbythebay.com/

https://linktr.ee/dianewaye YouTube **@stretchingbythebay**

Bounce Back from Back Pain is Diane's hybrid program featuring transformative, real-time-interactive & online sessions.

Chapter Sixteen
Money, Money, Money
by Dr. Theresa L. Smith, D.C.

Most of my life was a struggle with money. I didn't grow up with money, and my family definitely didn't know how to keep money. There was always a struggle, always a lack of that mystical money. When I was a child, both of my parents worked full-time jobs. My Dad worked two jobs. I watched them work hard, only to have nothing but struggle with paying the bills, feeding us, and housing us. We never took vacations.

Early Experiences with Money:

I started cleaning and cooking at a very young age, eight years old. I remember looking in the cupboard many times and only seeing one can of food. We were very creative in how we ate. One winter, I didn't have a coat, and my dad took me to Bullocks to buy me a nice coat. I have no idea how he afforded it or what he didn't pay to get that for me.

I remember answering the phone, and bill collectors were looking for their payments. I remember lying about where my parents were to them. It was an awful feeling. I was raised not to lie yet told to lie to whoever was on the phone looking for their money.

Very confusing!

Developing a Negative Relationship with Money:

All of this background led me to believe I didn't deserve money. I shouldn't have money. Money must be for those that work harder, work smarter, anything but what I had seen growing up. So, I worked really hard and still, not enough money to thrive. Survive barely, but not thrive. There is a difference. I decided long ago I wanted to thrive, not just survive.

I thought money was pure evil; the church told me so. I bought into borrowing money as a way of life. Loans, credit cards, which led to never having enough as well. It is a challenge to keep up with the payments; the interest alone will drown a person's soul. And there is the attitude of, I deserve to have something nice, even when you can't afford it. And we do deserve it, just not the aftermath of the payments.

Rewiring My Relationship with Money:

I did a lot of work around money: clearings, meditations, affirmations, and spells. I looked inside myself, outside myself. And then one day, I found a way to re-wire my brain. It was magical. I didn't change myself. Not one thing. Money just started showing up. It showed up in checks, new patients coming in without any changes in what I was doing or who I was. And it has just gotten better from there.

Focusing on True Desires:

Now I am also focusing on my true desires. As I desire to have more, so I can do more in life. I deluded myself by not having a true goal, a true desire. Now I know that knowing exactly what I desire, what I require for myself is key to also gathering up abundance in all areas of life: emotional, mental, and the bank.

The Impact of Money on Health:

While you may not think that money health relates to this book, it truly does. The lack of money gives a person stress and anxiety. Fear and uncertainty as to what the future holds, how you can pay your bills, and keep a roof over your head and your family's heads. Money also equates to control or power in social settings, affecting personal relationships.

The relationship to money deeply affects your emotional, mental, and physical health. Struggling with money affects every cell in your body. An unhealthy attitude towards money creates depression, mental fatigue, and stress. This all takes a heavy toll on your body. This will age you faster than one can imagine.

When you have enough money, there is no stress affecting your emotional, mental, and physical health. One is able to afford whatever is required for optimal health: supplements, massage, body classes, organic food, as an example.

Embracing Abundance:

So, say yes, even when you have no idea how you will pay for whatever it is. Say YES! Then, focus on that desire. That's it. Just focus on the desire. Don't listen to that voice that tells you you can't have it, you don't deserve it, you don't whatever. Ignore that voice. Keep focusing on your true desires!

A Conversation with Money:

I sat down after a meditation one day and had a chat with money. I looked at money and told it what I thought about it. Money, you are the root of all evil. Money, you evade me, and I don't know why. I think that for many, you (money) go easily to them and not to me. There must be something wrong with me. I must not deserve money. I must not know enough to have money. Money, I really hate that others have you so easily, and I don't. Why? Why oh why won't you come to me? I have a red wallet, just like someone told me that if I have a red wallet, you (money) would come to me. I keep all the bills in order as well. I was also told that would attract you (money). And still, I'm a chiropractor, and I should make money. What the H***??????

Then I pretended to be money and look at me. I learned how money felt about me. Money said it is always available to me, money wants to be with me, to help me thrive. Money told me I am blocked to receiving, and I say no too much. Money said I do love you and want to have a wonderful relationship with you. I told money, I can't be happy without you and yet you still evade me? Money told me to be happy with all the small things in life, to keep focusing on my desires, and money will start showing up.

Objectively, I took this information and have done nothing but focus on my true desires. I have been present and appreciated all the small things in life, gratitude, and guess what? Money started showing up. Now, I am deciding to make more money so that I can have my desired reality come to life. It is exciting and inspiring.

The Power of Yes:

When you say no to something because you can't afford it, this has a deep effect on all the parts of your brain. Consciously, it makes you feel badly, depressed, singled out. Subconsciously, it makes why you don't have money, can't have money even stronger in your wired neurons. You say no, you can't afford something. And over and over again, in your life, you will prove to yourself you can't afford anything. The more you prove it, the more you believe this deception!

When I looked at my beliefs about money and learned they aren't true, it changed my relationship and my bank account. My bank accounts are happier, and so is my body, mind, and soul. I invite you to have a conversation with money, let it know what you think about it. Then let it share what it thinks about you. Observe, be neutral. It will change your world.

About Dr. Theresa L. Smith, D.C.

My interest in the healing arts began when I was in my 20s, and I took courses in reflexology and massage. However, I had a career in business and family plans to settle down. I thought I knew where I was going. Life changed, and I was inspired to take my interest in the healing arts further to become a chiropractor. It took me ten years to realize my dream to help others through chiropractic care and other healing modalities as I worked full-time and parented my child as a single mother. I opened my first office in Sierra Madre and then moved to Monrovia 15 years later.

Studying how to help people feel better has never stopped. Today, I offer a multidisciplinary approach to health care that represents a unique blend of cutting-edge practices and interventions that, in my own experience, has proven to be effective. I focus on the true roots of each patient's health problems – what is unique to their situation – and choose the right treatment or approach that will make a lasting difference.

And now, since scientific research shows a clear link between what you think and how you feel affects your physiology and life, I am so happy to offer you tools to rewire your thought patterns and improve your health and life. To your health and well-being!

Chapter Seventeen

Starting Over at 56: Exploring the World Solo-Style

By Mary Adams

What an honor and a privilege to have the gift of life and to have lived this long.

I am this little biological accident born through my mom's universal womb as Mary, floating around in outer space on a planet called Earth. As I look up at the stars realizing I am a speck of dust in a vast universe, I know that I am more than this little human life, more than a critter roaming around on this big rock.

I turned 56 this year, and it was a mind-blowing experience to realize how fast time is going by. I feel like I have time warped into another dimension, as my brain truly can't conceive that I am towards the end of my life.

My concept of time is a bit out of sync as I still feel the energy and vibrancy of a 17-year-old, and yet when I look in the mirror, I am stunned and shocked to see that older woman with gray hair and little wrinkles smiling back at me. I realize that someone new has taken the reflection of that young lady I am so used to looking at every day. It is time to get to know this new version of myself and help her grow older gracefully, helping her to be comfortable in her elder body and prepare for the changes that are to come.

I often have the experience of scrolling through Facebook's news feed and seeing a face that looks familiar but just can't place how I know them. I quickly realize it's a friend of mine from high school or a neighbor, and although they've aged gracefully they still look so shockingly different. It is certainly not my goal to stay young forever, but I have been so busy raising a family, working, keeping food on the table, and being a mom - that it just zoomed by too fast, and my biggest wish is for just a little more time. I understand now that there is a gift in aging, and having the opportunity for that full spectrum long life, human experience is rare. From a little baby to an old lady, I feel like I won the golden ticket!

I am so grateful that I was born a woman, surrounded by a family that loved me and filled with matriarchs that were strong, stoic figures. They were powerful in their stature and grace, yet amongst the most gentle humans I have ever met. I was taught how to be a "proper young lady" and submit in a world where women were not equal to men. Growing up in the 70s was an interesting time of contrast, watching the growth of the women's equality movement on our black and white TV at 5 pm every night. It was the breaking of generational rules for our family in a new land to my ancestors, called America. Tradition and "old school" beliefs were important life messages and lessons guiding my future and choices.

I trusted them and was aware that they would never steer me wrong, and yet I was raised to believe that my job as a woman was to go to school, marry a good provider with skills and financial potential, settle down, and have kids. Watching my grandmothers, aunts, and mother in their daily routine had me brainwashed to believe that housekeeping and cooking were on my list of womanly duties while simultaneously working full time, tending to a family, keeping my man "happy," and tracking an accurate grocery list. There is a long line of ladies behind me and in front of me that have changed the definition of what it means to be a female on earth during the fast-paced transition and transformation for our gender. I am grateful for every woman who has broken the mold with hard work and sacrifices for the good of all. We have fought hard for opportunities that women in previous generations never had. We must cherish these advancements and hold onto them dearly, as our foremothers worked hard and diligently to raise the bar up to higher levels of equality. It is not ours to compete with the masculine society for control or power but to become more deeply connected to our own genuine femininity.

I grew up in Los Angeles and the lifestyle had me believing that the game of being successful had everything to do with how you show up in the world. The fat bank accounts and flashy bling with the race against time to buy the McMansion, and the new shiny car parked in the driveway, with two perfect kids. I played that game hard and followed all the rules. I shopped at the right stores with the popular brands, I said all the right things, and I behaved perfectly with the great grace and style of a modern L.A. businesswoman. I made sure to fit into the societal norms of my environment and stick to those etiquette lessons that I had been raised to adhere to.

"Elegance not flashy, preppy not trashy" was my life motto! At 22 years old, I landed a big corporate job, made "The Big Money," and bought the white picket fence and the whole Shabang. I did it all: I found the perfect husband, gave birth to 3 beautiful and amazing kids, Girl Scout Leader, and "Suzy Homemaker ''. I razzled and dazzled, had perfect holidays, and worked hard to be the ideal mother and queen of everything to my family and everyone else. It was a blessing to raise a family, and I most certainly was growing up right along with them. The satisfaction that I felt was a blessing, and yet I was rambling farther away from myself, forgetting what was important for me in this lifetime and who I really was inside. Parenting and marriage were a huge learning curve and with it so many tests and lessons to learn. What I know now is love is and always was the answer, and what is not love, never will be. Real love is not what we see in the movies or in those romance novels. I'm talking about that deep down-to-your-socks kind of love, the unconditional kind where you are 100% allowing that person to be who they are to their core. In complete acceptance not competition, and that we care for our partner with respect and individuality. Unconditionally supporting them to live their best life in their own way and to follow their dreams.

Our planet would be a different environment if we approached love, marriage, and family with a consciousness of how to be in a healthy relationship. The current dating and "hookup" culture does not afford us the opportunity to look consciously, to find out if we are a good match with our significant other. Being complimentary for sexual negotiations is not a good foundation to begin a lifelong commitment, and there is certainly nothing wrong with this aspect of a consensual relationship. But after the deed is done, the real foundation and truth of the connection is often meaningless and based on an afterglow rather than true love.

I have been divorced for 19 years and have had a few serious relationships, and it just never clicked or worked out the way my fantasy had promised. I have met plenty of nice guys with potential, and the love never sparked into anything bigger I realized that what I was looking for was rare, and up until now, solo life has been a more peaceful option. I had been sold the fairy tale of the princess at the ball, finding her prince charming, and everyone lived happily ever after … Now I know I have to create my own personal fairytale and my own happy ending.

This year, I became an official, newly certified, solo empty nester! My three daughters are successfully out in the world - 2 got married, and the youngest moved into her first place. They are busy with college, careers, husbands/partners, and full-time lives. If they could see themselves through my eyes, they would truly know how proud I am of each of them and I am cheering them on. It has taken me a while to get used to this chapter, coming to a close. I often reminisce about days gone by and I think of them all of the time. They were my life and my responsibility for almost 30 years, and now it's just me and the dogs.

No one told me that liquid love would leak out of my eyes from time to time when I think of them or that there would be moments of feeling such a big loss. I love them more than anything in the world, and they always have an open door and open arms with me. I am giving them that love, with wings to fly. Family is not replaceable, and they are the closest connection to you. Keep them near, cherish the time you have, and appreciate them for their uniqueness. Friends are chosen for things in common; family is your foundation from your past to your future.

I recently realized that I had never lived alone, not since my birth. There has always been another person living in the same vicinity and it's been a huge adjustment living in this big empty echoing house alone.

The first six months brought me to my knees. I missed my family and was so lost in not knowing how I was going to begin a new life without them. Deep loneliness and depression were the overtones of my days, and my sadness about feeling left behind to fend for myself had me feeling lifeless. I felt lost at moments, as my children were my reason for living and my "why" every day. They were my true motivation for living.

For months, I stayed home 24/7 waiting and hoping they would need me and I would be ready to jump up and be of service if one of them called. I could put on my super mom cape and spring into action, orchestrating their solution. But my phone rarely rang, and time passed by in silence and I had shut myself into the old life habits and routine that were holding me captive. I had no interest in looking beyond the confines of what I had created as my locked cell. I felt like a prisoner serving a life sentence. Holidays, birthdays, and outings were spent alone, and the big game changer for me was deciding not to waste any more time waiting.

I subconsciously was hoping that everything would go back to the way it was, everybody would come back home, and we could get back to normal. Then reality set in, and I was pushing hard against the truth so I could stay safe from the boogie monsters of grief. I had no idea what I wanted or what direction to head in. What I did not expect was to hit rock bottom after all of these years of successfully maneuvering through the world. I had to find the answer to pull myself out of the well of sadness that I had fallen into.

I am so grateful for my family and friends that extended a hand, a hug, or a word of comfort during this "dark night of the soul." Their wisdom and relatedness to my loss were comfort and confirmation that I would survive this chapter of my life. Their advice and guidance truly helped me understand and see a glimmer of hope for the future and gave me the courage to take the first steps towards my transformation. I started with simple baby steps to reclaim myself. A huge need for me in the beginning of this journey was just to be in pure silence. No one talking to me, begging, asking, pleading, demanding anything of me. To have my own thoughts, and to be able to follow through with the task of taking care of me, 100%. I was so conditioned to perform the caregiver role that I did not know how to truly take care of just me. In the midst of this journey, I was shocked and saddened to find out that "this" dear sweet woman inside had been living in survival mode most of her life, extinguishing all of the little fires daily for over five decades. It was a total game-changer for me! Here was my opportunity and reward after 30 years of parenting and raising children to finally be able to use the bathroom without interruption, finish a phone call, or watch a favorite documentary from beginning to end. These seem like such small and insignificant goals, and yet my life conformed to my family's needs. Who was I, and where do I find her again?

My BIG aha moment and breakthrough that changed everything came at 2:34 am on a typical Thursday early morning, after another night of practicing being a full-time insomniac.

My inner voice explained to me that "this was the first time in my life that I could do anything I wanted."

However, I wanted

Wherever I wanted

For as long as I wanted

With whomever I wanted

I know that sounds crazy, right?

But here's the truth, how many of us have gotten the opportunity to really do that for ourselves?

I looked at my bucket list, and I've added a lot of dreams and goals for my "retirement time" through the years. As I filter through them now, I'm not certain that they fit me anymore. Some of them are like 20-year-old outfits that are no longer in style, that ride up a little bit in the wrong place and are faded and worn thin. Reviewing and letting go of those old goals has been a necessary task to make room for the new life I am creating. To start over in a new direction, I needed to learn how to play "imagination games" again. I had not dreamed of a new life in a long time, and frankly, the thought of a fresh start after all of these years was frightening. I headed out into the world with new eyes looking for where my inspiration guided me, trying on new "life" scenarios to see how they fit.

I asked myself numerous questions and journaled the answers so I could get to the core of my own voice and choices.

What did this new version of me want?

How did she want to show up for herself?

Where did she want to be?

What created excitement for me?

What is on my MUST list before I die?

For the first time in my life, I have the independence to truly do a lot of what I want without interruption or permission. That fact

Navigating Wrinkles, Spasms and Generational Chasms

changed everything for me. I could decorate my home 100% with my flair and sass! My living space was finally my personal sanctuary and I now set the vibration and tone that I want. What a concept. Right?

I got to choose who and when someone was invited into my space and decide when I needed to ask them to leave and shut the curtains, lock the door, and nest inside. Through this process, I have been purging and getting rid of so much unneeded "Stuff" … mentally, physically, emotionally, and spiritually. And tending to the undoing, unbecoming, unfolding, and getting to the core of who I am. It has been worth the effort and time that I have dedicated to doing my deep work and birthing into the next version of me.

I have learned so many lessons about myself along the way and what is important to me:

1. Choose what fills you up and nurtures you.

    Be satisfied with what you have and discard what messes with that.

    Choose peace in your home, environment, and relationships, and you will have more peace in your life.

2. Be keen and pay attention to everything you are choosing for yourself.

    Is what you are choosing in alignment with your beliefs, future, lifestyle, and soul?

    We unknowingly make 1,000's of decisions every day… are they serving you?

    Are they nurturing and feeding you, or are they even the right frequency?

3. Honor yourself in every way you can and be kind to you.

    We have a tendency to be damaging and critical with

ourselves out of habit and self-abuse. The overthinking and trying to change what's behind you will get you nowhere. When you feel stuck there are always options, even when you can't see it right away.

4. Nothing is usually as serious as we make it out to be.

   Life happens "Things stop working", mistakes pop up and plans crash down. I remember having moments through my life that confused and frustrated me, because it was not happening my way, my chosen outcome. Learn to let go!

5. Throw that rearview mirror into the garbage can and stop dragging those heavy chains of your past behind you.

   Move forward and look ahead of you. Pay attention to where you are going.

6. You are more powerful than you will ever know.

   Limitations are taught to us and indoctrinated into us. We have been conditioned as women to play small and follow the rules.

I want to remind you that you have your brilliance, your wisdom, and your beautiful mind. It knows the answers, and the next step is to listen to yourself. Don't be afraid to shine too brightly or jump too high. When you find something that inspires you and ignites you from within, that is the direction to go. Dream bigger - contemplate deeper and think broader and wider. Put your energy and your heart into your new life, and you will reap the rewards of the happiness and contentment that you crave. Owning yourself as a powerful woman is not boasting or being selfish. It is the confidence and grace of a woman who knows her worth.

The new life: I am enjoying my own company, dancing with the dogs in the kitchen at 2 am with the music turned up loud, singing, and carrying on. I take myself out on dates and explore the world solo style. My life is in creation mode as I am finishing up two diploma programs, writing books, and exploring new career options that excite me and ignite me. My home has become my sanctuary and place of comfort and peace. No more tight clothes, ugly furniture, or humans that have funky energy. Anything that doesn't make me feel great is out the door. I am becoming someone new at every moment as I enter this last phase of my life. I am claiming it and jumping back into the deep end of being the true feminine human that I am and allow the gentle essence of me to reemerge with the sweetness that I was born with. I want my innocence back, and I have made a vow to myself to find it as I look through each layer of my being. I am ripping off the conditioning, brainwashing, and toughened-up masculine attitude that I had to take on to maneuver and survive through this crazy world. I allow myself to be soft and flowing, reigniting my freedom to play and reclaim my inner child. It has been a learning process to trust myself fully and let my womanly wisdom be my guide. So that I may become who I truly am and was and always meant to be. The feeling of completeness fills me as I do the deep discovery to find the hidden gems of my mind, human body, and soul. There are insights and healing within each step as another layer lifts off of me. I feel a deep sense of freedom and blessed to be blooming. I choose to live on purpose, with my life moments lived purposefully.

My creation is unfolding as my final masterpiece; I have reclaimed my life and built a new story for myself. What a gift that is!

The biggest lesson I have learned about this life is that you just never know when it's your time to go. I often ask myself the question, "If I were to leave this planet today, would I have done everything that I came here to do?" My current answer is a big NO. I have people to see and thank for a wonderful life, and those last hugs and tender moments with my parents, kids, family, and friends are at the top of my list. I hope we get the gift of watching each other grow old. I want to spread all the good that I can and leave my thumbprint of kindness upon this earth.

I am not running towards the end of my life or running away from it, but filling these last chapters of my story with importance and meaning is a high priority for me.

When my time comes, and we have to say goodbye.

To my family, friends, and loved ones:

Your kindness and love have been the guiding light on my journey, I am grateful for our connection and memories. I love you with every fiber in my being and I am grateful that we had the opportunity to cross paths in this life. Please remember the good times, the laughter, and the celebrations.

To my daughters:

You have shown me a love that I never knew existed, and being your mother has been the grand prize of this life. Your time here is a miracle and be sure to live it to its fullest and, experience it all, and be alive in every way you can. My love for you is beyond space and time, a bond that can never be broken. I will be with you for eternity, watching over you. Feel my embrace when you call out for me and listen for my whispers in your ear. Thank you for being my greatest teachers and the deepest loves of my life. I will forever cherish our time together; you are my greatest blessings.

Mom, Mama Bunny, and Dad:

Thank you for giving me the gift of life and every moment, every sacrifice, and truly being present for me every day in every way. I love you, and our strong friendship and family ties have been the guiding force throughout my life. You have been on this path with me through it all, always ready to help and love me through it. I am grateful to each of you for our special bond and connection. Keep me in your heart, and I will always be with you. I love you.

I am so grateful for the lessons of this life. The good, the bad, the happy, the sad. Being a human is a tough assignment, and if there is anything that did not sit right between us, I hope you can forgive me. For me, there are no grudges, no bad feelings, and nothing left unsaid. My truth is that who I have become, who I have grown into, what I have experienced, triumphed, failed at, overcome, and risen above is my celebration of this well-lived life. I got the opportunity to do it all! I am so proud that I lived this life out loud, adventure girl, blazing the trail, brave and strong when others would run. I danced wildly, I sang at the top of my lungs, I loved with an open heart, and I climbed the mountains and swam in the sea.

Find me in the sunset, find me in the sea, I will love you forever, for you belonged to me.

About Mary Adams

Mary Adams is a published Best Selling author, dreamer and facilitator, who is passionate about empowering others to their highest potential. She is owner of "Infinity Global Creations" A Promotion and Marketing Firm, Established in 2008 - She enjoys working with best selling authors, rising stars and famous musicians, to expand their audiences for marketing, products and social media globally. infinityglobalcreations.com

Chapter Eighteen

The Pause: After All, I Am Still 'Hot' - Just in Flashes Now

by Claudia Micco

It can definitely be brutal.

The "Pause" showed up right on time. In January 2018, after my 51st birthday, I noticed the telltale signs of my last period. I won't go into too much detail, but it was a slow drip to the last drop, and being hypersensitive to my body and its messages, I knew that was it. My body felt different, lighter, almost like a weight had been lifted. A slight grin spread across my face as I realized my timing was impeccable, according to most statistics. Finally, an A+ on this test - menopause at 51! The monthly ritual of cramps, cravings, blood, and gore, among other things, had come to an end. For decades, it ruled the majority of my life, dictating when and how I could do things. Each month brought relief when it arrived, but I always knew that it would no longer come one day, and I would be free from its messy burden. I had an agreement with puberty that this relationship would have an expiration date. For me, it was like being freed from a never-ending subscription to a crappy magazine. I was shedding my old skin for older crepey skin, but nonetheless, I would be stepping into a new phase of life. I remember naively thinking, "Oh well, at least now I can officially say goodbye to those dreadful days and embrace this new phase of life"... if only my body would cooperate.

The aging of a woman, you know, the "Pause," formerly known as "The Grand Pause," to signify the pause button pressed on certain bodily functions at a certain age, with various other terms such as "The Change of Life," our secret little rite of passage into some new phase of existence, and another fun one, Climacteric, which comes from the Greek word "klimakter," meaning "critical point," which imparts a sense of gravity as if menopause were a cosmic event akin to the alignment of planets. Any name you give it, it's not exactly a topic most people like to discuss. Maybe it's because our mothers never told us about it, or perhaps they didn't want to scare us. I would have preferred something more akin to "the vagina dialogues" - because, let's be real, our mothers didn't exactly sit us down for a chat about it. But now, as we embrace the changes of aging, it becomes a necessary dialogue about what it means to be a woman in this new stage of life and the unexpected head-shaking experiences that come with it. Who knew going through "the change" would require so much...well, change? The conversation about vaginas, well, sort of, continues...

I thought entering menopause would bring a sense of freedom, but instead, it brought unexpected challenges. As a mind-body fitness instructor who always emphasized physical, mental, and spiritual well-being, I thought I was prepared for this change. I had been working out and teaching for over 30 years, and I honestly thought it would be a few hot flashes, a quick change of my sheets, and back to business as usual. Ironically, I never even had too many hot flashes. Who knew menopause would be more like a hot mess than a hot flash? The physical changes in my body were gradual, almost imperceptible at first. Wrinkles forming at the corners of my eyes and mouth, hints of gray in my hair, and a softening of my muscles. But overall, I still felt and looked like myself.

But that all changed during a business trip to Australia; while teaching Yoga workshops and creating unforgettable memories with my students, I was unexpectedly hit with my period as I approached my 52nd birthday. Of course, it had to happen on the final day of the trip when I was wearing my favorite white and black yoga pants. The experience was a rollercoaster of emotions - happiness, connection, embarrassment, and surprise - as my body went through unexpected changes during what seemed like a perfect moment. Thankfully, my students were understanding and even found humor in the situation. "Let's take a break from downward dogs." "Who can run to the pharmacy and grab some tampons?" "Do you need a change of clothes?" "Might as well get me some chocolate while you're at the pharmacy." Although it was funny in hindsight, I was initially mortified. Who would have thought that periods could make a surprise attack on us after we thought they were long gone? It's like playing an endless game of hide-and-seek with our bodies. Imagine teaching a workshop and suddenly feeling like you're bursting a water balloon. Don't look down! There was a distinct scent to this new phase of my life - a mix of sweat and fear - as I faced unknown challenges ahead. The sound of my body adjusting to these changes is a constant hum, or rather, like Snap, Crackle, Pop - the old Rice Krispies providing background music to remind me that I am no longer in complete control of every aspect of my physical being.

In the past, women remained silent about The Pause, which sounds like a better name for an alternative rock band. It was a taboo topic, on par with Voldemort in terms of how it was spoken of - not at all. It was seen as a personal and private issue, off-limits for open discussion. Limited education and lack of access to information about women's health kept many in the dark about their bodies. Women were supposed to stick to domestic duties and bear any discomfort stoically, like a champ. I don't know, but maybe some women didn't even suffer from symptoms, or they were just too busy running the household to notice. Even the medical community was uninformed, only studying menopause later in the 20th century. I am sure they were too busy studying other matters like baldness cures or creating new ice cream flavors and penis enlargers. This lack of knowledge and resources contributed to a sense of secrecy and isolation within society. The topic of menopause and perimenopause carried a scent of shame and secrecy that mingled with the floral scents of women's beauty products and household cleaners. During this time, women were expected to maintain appearances and uphold a certain level of "feminine" hygiene. Special products, like FDS: Feminine Deodorant Spay, masked any natural odors "down there," including those associated with menopause and perimenopause. Women were left in ignorance, unable to fully comprehend or embrace their bodies, while society and the medical community ignored their struggles. Thankfully, things are shifting in a more positive direction. We can openly discuss mood swings and the hidden nuances of menopause beyond the hot flash without feeling embarrassed or like we're divulging forbidden knowledge. Thank you, society, for allowing us women to speak openly about our hormonal farewell.

The physical toll of aging can be unrelenting, brutal even at times. I have always relied on my body to make a living; it is basically my business card. Despite being in an industry obsessed with youth, ego, and muscles, I kept it together pretty well over the years. But as the years have passed, I've noticed changes in myself and my female clients. The bitter pill of acceptance, as I come to terms with the fact that the muscles in my arms now have visible wrinkles, and can we talk about the loose skin? My fingers trace over the creases and folds, a reminder of the naked truth of time's grip on my body. The once ostentatious display of my body may not fare well in the face of limitations and inability, forcing me to confront the naked truth of my mortality. My clients, too, have to accept the changes in their bodies. But it's a version of reality we face together. I've come to love the physical changes that come with age. Truly a delightful experience. At least we can bond over our shared confusion.

For instance, although my clients lived healthy lifestyles or were former athletes, as they aged, they all started to experience increased discomfort in their muscles and bones without a clear explanation. I've sent many of them for various tests - MRIs, bloodwork, you name it - but nothing ever produced a definitive answer. There were always missing pieces to the puzzle. After extensive research over the years, I discovered that the decline of estrogen levels in our bodies can lead to subtle changes in tissue, resulting in persistent pain. Although it is widely known that estrogen plays a significant role in women's sexual health, regulating sex drive, vaginal well-being, and fertility. What isn't discussed so much is that it also affects other bodily functions such as bone density, brain function, muscle strength, and heart health. Having low estrogen levels can make you feel "weird," causing an overall feeling of unease. Sometimes, it's hard to pin down what exactly feels off.

As if hot flashes and mood swings weren't enough for women, the decrease in estrogen during perimenopause and menopause wreaks havoc on muscle tissue, bones, and ligaments. This change affects every muscle in the body, from head to toe. It is something to behold. The creaking of aging joints and muscles echoes in the room, a symphony, the sound of groans and sighs as the body struggles to move. The loss of estrogen leads to higher cortisol levels, resulting in tension and pain throughout the body's muscles. Even the often-overlooked pelvic floor muscles may be impacted, causing dysfunction and discomfort for many women.

But who needs strong and well-developed muscles anyway? Oh, right...we do. Muscle stem cells, also known as satellite cells, are a specific type of stem cell found in muscle tissue. They play a critical role in repairing and rebuilding skeletal muscles. Estrogen is essential for regulating the function of these cells and maintaining their health. During menopause, estrogen levels decline, causing muscle stem cells to decrease in number, resulting in a reduced ability for the body to repair and regenerate muscle tissue. This can lead to noticeable changes in our bodies, such as a sagging butt or flabby muscles. The term "flabby assed" must have originated from this phenomenon. Tackling these changes during menopause requires a comprehensive approach that includes lifestyle adjustments, regular exercise, and possibly medical interventions.

The "Pause" is no joke; it can be a real buzzkill, but it is more fun to make jokes about it and have a good time. Now, let me give you some words of wisdom I've lived by - first things first, move your body and exercise. You don't have to kill yourself doing it. There are ways to stay in shape and keep your sanity intact. Don't worry. My clients and I have found success with a combination of weightlifting, cardio, walking, pilates, and yoga to keep ourselves in shape. We joke about going from an hourglass figure to a triangular one during menopause, but any shape is healthy if you care for your body. I mean, who doesn't love a good geometric makeover? The key is to find something you actually enjoy doing. Consistently exercising is tough enough without dreading it every time. I won't lie; my mood swings are more than just minor annoyances; they can range from feeling grateful for my long and amazing life to wondering how my ego will handle having more years behind me than ahead of me. But hey, at least I'm still here. Excuse me while I walk off this mood swing.

As I enter this stage of post-menopause, my body is hosting a grand finale party with all the classic symptoms and some unexpected ones. The Pause feels like a never-ending gift that keeps on giving. Did you know estrogen plays a crucial role in brain function by aiding blood flow and neurotransmitter activity? Those feel-good chemicals that were once connecting are changing. Then, as estrogen levels decrease, irritability, poor concentration, forgetfulness, and exhaustion occur. This can create a sense of "brain fog" and make daily activities more challenging, including exercise. But do it anyway. You are only one workout away from a better mood. While my hormones are still on a seesaw, I'm preparing for some interesting times ahead. Say goodbye to a sharp memory because who needs it? I've become an expert at charades, perfecting my skills while trying to communicate with others. Who needs exact words when you have exaggerated hand gestures and facial expressions? Every day feels like a game of Password or Pictionary. My friends and I are getting quite inventive with our acting skills - we might even start an improv group—the Pause Players. So yes, menopause may be challenging, but it's definitely keeping us entertained.

Is it essential to embrace the aging process for one's mental well-being? Yes, that's what I'm supposed to say. Of course, who wouldn't want to look like a raisin with wrinkles and age spots in a society that values youthfulness? Most of us know estrogen plays a role in keeping skin supple and hydrated by producing sebum and collagen;

when that starts to go down, so does the skin. However, I can't help but long for my youthful and smooth skin. I was fortunate until I wasn't. When I first noticed my skin becoming thinner and crepe-like, I almost fell out of my rocking chair—all those years of surfing and tanning drenched in baby oil mixed with iodine finally caught up to me in my 50s. No amount of yoga, positive thinking, or creams and exfoliants can reverse that damage. It seems like my options are either finding a partner who doesn't mind sensory deprivation during sex or one with poor eyesight for a chance at lasting love. But perhaps we should embrace our natural aging process and all the wisdom that comes with it - after I slather on some anti-aging cream and do a face mask, of course.

Are you constantly anxious about the changes in your once perky and youthful breasts? Don't worry; have faith that they can still maintain some semblance of their former glory, if you're lucky, that is. Only one in five women experience an increase in breast size after menopause, and the most significant factor associated with this change is weight gain. Unfortunately, I can't rely on that option as I have never had to pay much attention to my breasts before. They were always a source of pleasure for me with their "perfect for me" size and shape. My previous partner even joked that anything more than a handful was too much for him to handle. But then menopause hit, transforming my feminine curves into what felt like pecs. Man boobs? I never even considered that possibility. Now, I can't help but wonder if they would even be considered bite-size anymore. And don't get me started on certain sexual positions; being on top has become a mental challenge, especially with the lights on. It's like playing mental gymnastics with lighting and body positioning to avoid looking down. Ironically, despite these changes, I am now more aware and in tune with my body and its desires compared to when I was younger. My libido still matches that of a teenager, but with a completely different physique, and yes, it does get thinner "down there," too. This is the other thing that seems to slim down without dieting. That's why it's vital to keep lube by the bedside. Yes, even the vagina changes as we age - not just in thickness and color but also in smell, as acidity levels decrease a little bit, among other things. This change can be confusing and embarrassing to talk about, but it's entirely normal and isn't a bad thing. It serves as a reminder of the natural aging process and how society's narrow beauty standards and desirability no longer align with our bodies. Perhaps gracefully aging means accepting these inevitable changes and embracing our uniqueness. And, of course, regular self-exams and mammograms are still crucial. Even though my girls may have regressed from voluptuousness to prepubescent knobs, I will never miss my mammogram appointments. After all, it's often the only action they get nowadays.

The Pause can be tricky, with mood, physical changes, and cultural shifts making things even more interesting. As someone with a lot of life experience, I've learned not to care too much about what others think so much anymore. I am part of that secret society now, the one who rolls their eyes at young people baking in the sun and understands the irony behind it. I try to focus on my path, but as a member of Generation X, I am still constantly surprised by the changes in society. The "Karens" we knew were just Karen Carpenter's sweet singing voice; now they're entitled customers yelling at innocent baristas. It's surreal to think that in such a short amount of time, women have gained and lost control over their bodies. Powerful anthems like Helen Reddy's "I Am Woman" still hold true today - "I know too much to go back and pretend." Despite all the cultural shifts, I still believe our generation had the best music. But seeing so many of my favorite artists pass away is bittersweet. Each feels like a personal loss like an old friend leaving this world without saying goodbye. It's like one big cosmic joke - when we finally have enough life experience to truly appreciate their lyrics, they're no longer around to sing them.

And yes, while advancements in medicine have allowed us to go on HRT and allow people with HIV to live longer and healthier lives, I can't help but think about what could have been for my friends who didn't make it. In my 20s, many of my close friends died from HIV. They were young, handsome, and full of life, taken too soon by a tragic illness that was misunderstood and stigmatized at the time. But there is still a lingering sadness when I think about what their futures could have held. In my memories, they will always be frozen in time - forever young and vibrant. Who knows what kind of trouble and mischief we could have gotten into as old folks? The reality of death hits harder now, as it reminds me of its inevitability and the fragility of all life.

As I look towards my uncertain future, I can't help but acknowledge the changes that come with aging. My body and mind are no longer immune to the inevitable alterations that time brings. Who would have thought that even pubic hair could turn grey? And the thought of potentially needing a pessary is both daunting and surreal. It's a constant reminder that my perception of myself will inevitably shift as I age. And if I am fortunate enough to reach old age, the memories that people hold of me may not reflect the image I see in the mirror - instead of a young and fit woman, they may see an older, wrinkled woman more learned. No longer am I the carefree and youthful figure I once was. But in exchange, I hope to become a wiser and more experienced version of myself. It's strange yet humbling to consider how time can profoundly alter our perspectives and memories.

Ah, the surprises of growing old. Despite all the unexpected changes, one thing is certain: empathy, patience, and humor are essential in navigating this journey. After all, I now understand firsthand the advice I used to give my clients in my younger years. Whether it's hot flashes or gravity taking its toll on our bodies, we must stick together and embrace renewal at any age. Here's to making it past 50. The irony is not lost on me. Aging is truly a hilarious adventure - my arm keeps waving long after I've stopped, gravity is no longer my friend, and I've made it to this age by the skin of my thighs. After all, I am still "hot" - just in flashes now.

About Claudia Micco:

Claudia Micco, a renowned fitness trainer from Maui, blends yoga, Pilates, and hypnosis in her transformative HypnoFitness method. An author of the best-selling book "Lessons Learned the Hard Way," she's also a respected speaker and contributor to CanFitPro and other publications, advocating for holistic health and trauma-sensitive training globally. Learn more at www.claudiamicco. com

Chapter Nineteen
Tech Neck (R): The Pandemic That's Steadily Hurting Our Women
by Gregory Kirschenbaum, LMT

In a world where men rule almost everything and women Do almost everything, we find ourselves in a unique social schema. But that's only where it starts. As a man in holistic medicine, most days, I find myself at odds with this schema. It doesn't make any physical, spiritual, or medical sense. The type of medicine I practice is fully integrative. I'm a different type of Licensed Massage Therapist. I practice internal medical massage and Traditional Chinese Medicine. I am also a successful Energy Medicine Provider. This goes so far beyond a spa rub down or Reiki. This is the type of therapy where you actually get better. Your pain goes away with me because I get to the truth of your disease or disorder.

Who will come to see me? Post-Pandemic…practically, everyone. Women lead the way by a ratio of something like 8:1. Of course, there are always a few smart men who know to come for therapy, but this is about the 8, not the 1. There is a definite need for the men to come in for manual (and mental health) therapy as well, but it is the women who tend to "do the work" and find themselves in a positive direction with one or more therapists.

Thank God.

After more than 30 years of either certified or licensed physical therapeutic touch on a patient, I have noticed all types of patterns. What is most common among the women in America?

Neck, back, and hip pain. And then, there's the tummy…

Let's start with the Neck and work our way down the body.

About 10 years ago, I was running the Massage Therapy part of Spear Physical Therapy in NYC. They are basically, the largest private PT group in NYC. We were busy. One day, I was having lunch with the Clinic Director, and he asked me about "Mrs. Johnson" (we'll use an anonymous name to protect the patient's privacy). I replied, "She's one powerful lady. She'll keep that money machine turning for her and her family, but that 'TECH NECK' will probably never go away. All I'll ever be able to do for her is help her manage it and hopefully, prevent it from becoming even more progressive."

He said, "Her what???"

I quipped, "What? Her Tech Neck?"

He immediately wrote it down and asked, "Can we use that phrase?"

A decade later, everyone pretty much knows the basic concept of "Tech Neck."

Since that day in the clinic when I had my "Reese's peanut butter cup moment" and blurted out the name of this disorder, I've discovered a whole lot more about it than just neck pain. Of course, it's progressive. Meaning if and when left untreated, Tech Neck advances through the Central Nervous System (CNS) to the Peripheral Nervous System (PNS: Arms, Legs, Hands, Feet, Fingers, and Toes), thus creating all sorts of problems for the person. This is not only limited to radiating down the body. It can also travel up the neck, to the jaw, and certainly, to the rest of the skull. This may cause you to grind your teeth, clench your jaw at the TMJ (Temporal Mandibular Joint) and absolutely create things like Tinnitus, earaches, blurred or disturbed vision, sinus, tension, occipital, ocular, and even migraine headaches.

Let's go back down the head back to the neck. I mentioned the word "occipital" or Occiput. That is the round notch at the base of our skull, where the top of the vertebral column meets the skull. The neck, or cervical spine, is stacked with seven vertebrae and lots of other soft tissue to hold us all together. This isn't an anatomy lesson, but I do want to make sure everyone gets a taste of just how complicated Tech Neck can be.

At the Occiput, the cervical spine meets the skull and supports that 12-lb. "Bowling Ball" that runs our Lives. Inside that skull is obviously, our brain, the central nervous system's main computer. Directly inferior (below) the brain is the brain stem and the spinal cord. These three parts of the body comprise the entire central nervous system. I include the brain stem as a separate component of the CNS. Other medical professionals prefer to combine the brain and brain stem into one component, so they'll describe the CNS as having just two aspects: the brain and spinal cord. I like the three because the brain stem produces stem cells which go on to differentiate later in the cellular process of the body, thus creating the rest of the body. So, I feel it deserves its own componentry.

Off the spinal cord are lots and lots more nerves. They go everywhere in our bodies. The Peripheral nervous system (PNS remember) is highly affected by the compression that occurs at the neck. That's the basic issue with Tech Neck. The Cervical Spine becomes compressed through postural decay. Meaning we sit at the computer, on the phone, or even in teleconferencing and flex the neck forward while holding that 12lb skull, out of proper postural position. The result…Neck Pain.

Which then travels. Up or down. Once it does migrate down, there's an entire body for it to attack. Neck to Shoulder is typically first. The tops of our shoulders (the "Traps") tend to be most common. They become either hard as a rock or develop that

"Ball" inside the muscle. Commonly called, "Knots", they are actually Trigger Points. Discovered, researched, and taught by the incomparable Dr. Janet Travell, Trigger Points is an enormous "thing" in physical neuromuscular medicine. I don't have the space here to get deeper into it now, but I urge you to go down a rabbit hole about this when you have time. Very often, Trigger Points IS THE REASON for your radiating pain. Thank you Dr. Travell for teaching us all this very important part of Physiology. She absolutely deserves all the respect and appreciation possible. We are all better because of her and her work.

Back to the Traps. The trapezius is one large broad back muscle that attaches at the neck and goes all the way down to the Sacrum! There really is no such thing as "Upper – Middle – nor Lower" Traps. It's all one contiguous muscle. As such, it contains a network of nerves. It, along with every single muscle in our body, is wrapped with a neuro-fibrous material known as "Fascia". This wraps the muscle AND the muscle group and holds everything together as well as sends signals through the entire area (as well as the whole body). This is part of the reason why I and many others maintain that to treat any one aspect of our body, we can look at the entire body as a whole. Holistic Medicine should be renamed "WHOLISTIC MEDICINE."

The Trap and all of the back muscles are connected to all of the posterior nerves emanating from the Spinal cord itself. These nerves then follow the rest of the body down the arms, wrists and fingers. Same dynamic. Fascia wraps the muscles and the muscle groups. Then the nerves all connect to the entire region. The compression that started up at the neck now sends either restricted or compromised nerve signals to the shoulders, back, arms, wrists, and fingers. Then, the exact same thing can happen all the way down from the back to the lower body. Remember how the Traps attach to the sacrum? Well, there are a ton of nerves down there. Kinda like the way a tree has a ton of roots underground. All the branches of the tree are similar to our brains. The tree trunk; is our Spinal cord. The tree roots; are our sacral nerves. Then there's that one famous long nerve that runs down our leg and causes so much horror in the world. The Sciatic Nerve... Best known for causing "Sciatica".

Yes. Sciatica can easily be triggered by Tech Neck. Once it sets in, you will most likely need to go to a very well-trained therapist to get out of this type of pain. Many people experience Sciatic flare-ups. It is also very common from driving. I have paired sciatic pain to tech neck many times, but I've also coupled it with anxiety and depression as well. Very common for nerve and neuromuscular pain to arise from both.

Travel further down the body. Sciatic pain aside, let's talk about the feet.

Pedicures are great. I love them. I don't often get them, but every once in a while, I stop what I'm doing, drive over to a nice salon in the neighborhood, and walk in. I'm almost always the only man. And typically, in unison, there's a roomful of women who turn their heads to see who's walking in next and offer me a huge smile. Nary a one has ever uttered even a word. Just a sweet warm smile. I never tell anyone I'm a massage therapist. I just sit back and enjoy myself, like anyone would when they're getting a foot pampering.

That's the outside of the feet. Tech Neck will go all the way down the body to the internal aspect of the feet and cause ongoing chronic foot pain. The nerves get compressed at the lower back as well, not just the neck (it can definitely become like a domino effect in the vertebral column). Once the lower back becomes compressed, we're typically looking at some ongoing therapy. It usually means that you're dealing with some chronic pain. And that usually means that you have been at it for years!

There's an entire book coming about this. I will be diving really deeply into these waters. Tech neck actually transforms from a neuromuscular disorder into an Internal Organ disorder, causing acute and chronic disease. It can be said that Everything in the Body is Neurological. Once one part of the nervous system becomes compromised, any number of problems may occur. My career is focused on helping (women) out of acute and chronic pain. Over the past three decades, I have seen 1000s of people from all walks of life. The one thing that holds true for the vast majority of them is that they are living in acute and chronic pain brought on by Tech Neck, which evolved because they are sitting at the computer or on the phone a lot. This will ultimately, destroy the human body and create many different forms of pain, disorders, and ultimately internal organ damage and disease.

It's hard to be gorgeous, the best at work, and a great mom, wife, partner, daughter, sister, caregiver, teacher, nun, Goddess, therapist, animal rescuer, protector, advocate, doctor, confidant, repairwoman, disciplinarian, librarian, chief, cook, and bottle-washer.

Thank you for putting up with us men!

About Gregory Kirschenbaum, LMT:

Greg is a nationally recognized artist and medical Empath. Born and raised, a native New Yorker, he made his career first as an art director in global advertising, then as they say, got out of "jail" and pursued his painting and sculpting career. After working on the Ground Zero statues, "Lunchtime Atop a Skyscraper". His work became known by millions. But his true creative passion is composing music, painting and writing stories. Greg had many sides and after his heart attack at 44, he returned to school in NYC and earned a degree in massage therapy. He then stayed in school and has been pursuing his Masters and Doctorate in Traditional Chinese Medicine

Chapter Twenty
The Art of UNBECOMING

by Monica Rodgers

"Maybe the journey isn't so much about becoming anything. Maybe it's about un-becoming everything that isn't really you, so you can be who you were meant to be in the first place."

-Paul Coelho

At 53 years old, I am Unbecoming again, dissolving, growing, and morphing into yet another version of myself.

With any change, I have to remember to welcome the familiar wings of anxiety-like those that woke me this morning, first fluttering gently as I woke and then more forcefully as I prepared for the day.

I heard her question as I poured myself a cup of coffee.

"Is it safe to change?" she asked.

"Yes," I responded, reminding her that like a snake dropping its skin, I am shedding another layer to reveal the shiny vernix of a truer me as I surrender to another cycle of Unbecoming as I take a six-month self-imposed sabbatical to travel, draw and paint- to allow my inner artist self to be excavated and known.

Unbecoming is a transformative alchemy that has occurred in phases over the past 16 years, and I have come to trust where it takes me. The more I allow it, the more alive I become.

It began with a 'dark night of the soul' - a divorce and a health crisis that put me in bed for 9 months, but which ultimately saved my life. It was there that I discovered how to love myself and that I benefited from unraveling myself from the disempowering stories and lies that held me, prisoner in my own life.

Until then, I had been living someone else's version of my life. I was unconsciously yet relentlessly ruled by false "feminine" virtues that were shaping me into some future version of a Stepford wife or, at the very least, a cookie-cutter version of other girls my age. I learned to perform my role 'self' expertly, so much so that I forgot who I was beneath the insidious cultural conditioning.

To "grow up girl" meant I was corrected and redirected at every turn. From my earliest memory, I was rarely free from the adult gaze or the continual admonishments, edits, conditions, disapproval, or judgment of the adults around me.

It's unbecoming to sit that way - cross your legs, Monica!

It's unbecoming to be so boisterous! - settle down, Monica!

It's unbecoming to dress that way - don't draw attention to yourself, Monica!

It's unbecoming to be sexual- don't be a slut, Monica!

It's unbecoming to argue - go to your room till you can act right, Monica!

Slowly but surely, I put away the free-thinking, curious, artistic, adventurous, and boisterous parts of myself. I was aware of the freedoms afforded to boys and increasingly dismayed by the narrow confines of what it meant to be a girl in the world. I was flummoxed by why our options were so limited, while in contrast, the expansive opportunities and choices available to my brother made my blood boil.

When it came time to apply for college, my well-intentioned father told me, "You'll never find a husband who can provide for you in Art School." Despite the excitement and scholarships, I was to go to a liberal arts college, and there was no more talk of art school. I would do as he wished if I wanted financial support.

Like all "good girls," I learned to suppress my needs and desires. I learned to stuff it, and to say "yes" when I meant "no" and "no" when I meant "yes." I learned to "go along to get along," to turn on myself when I couldn't get it right and to pretend it didn't matter to me anyway.

Plagued by doubt and self-loathing, my perfectionist tendencies would eventually lead to body aches, migraines, and bouts of dark depression. In addition to prescription drugs and other vices, I began to self-medicate.

Meanwhile, the parts I had oppressed and denied, the parts of myself that were stifled, scorned, and betrayed, were locked away in the dank, dark cellar of my inner world, waiting for me to someday return.

I became a participant in the slow and steady erasure of Self, the dark but essential ritual of this world that requires us to bury the true Self alive - entombed within the feminine graveyard of patriarchy.

The parts of me that didn't belong—that were too much or not enough—were exiled and banished to places far away. So far, in fact, I might have lost them forever were it not for the tiniest spark within me that lay dormant, refusing to die. Indeed, somewhere inside me was The Little Match Girl, as I would see quick sparks of life and a woman I knew was me before the visions would swiftly burn out. Something else was revealing itself.

This type of resurrection, however, can only happen after a death of sorts. In my case, it was the death of the persona I had formed over all of those years - the identity of the "good girl" that I had created and fortified to survive an emotionally uninhabitable world.

The woman who was taught to forgo her own knowing and to find a nice husband, and a home with a white picket fence.

In a world that still persisted in defining the feminine as pretty, pleasing, and polite. I was also expected to be selfless, nurturing, obedient, compliant, responsible, modest, and physically perfect. I have yet to meet more than a few adult women who have escaped the slow and steady onboarding into "the trance of unworthiness."

Does this sound dramatic? It's not. From birth, females are micro-dosed messages that culminate over time into an inner cognitive hypnosis. Like Stockholm syndrome, we tend to acquiesce to our captors, eventually forgetting that we were ever free, and simply go about making our cage more comfortable.

While fully expressed in my early years as artistic, bold, sensitive, assertive, adventurous, imaginative, and highly curious, I was also considered bossy, rough, strong, fast, and dramatic.

Unfortunately, none of these qualities were encouraged, and I would soon learn to shut these aspects of myself away and to edit the parts deemed "unladylike" or "unbecoming" by the adults in my life.

While I tried to meet expectations, I struggled mightily to conform to the path that seemed paved for me, and try as I might, I was always getting into trouble.

Like an IV inserted at birth, negative messages permeated my psyche and were force-fed with a steady diet of diminishing returns. I was endlessly confused by the contradictions of what it meant to be female.

In surrender, I became who I thought my parents and teachers wanted me to be by silencing the parts of myself that were too naive, messy, loud, shiny, and opinionated. Alternately, I learned to overcompensate for my shortcomings by wearing masks to hide the parts that didn't belong.

Like wearing makeup, I learned to hide the blemishes and put on my game face—a shiny exterior veneer—hiding my true self away behind layers of deception. I got so good at it, I even fooled myself!

The phrase "fake it till you make it" became significant. I dedicated myself to winning at any cost, doubling down by perfecting my outward appearance and essentially living in ways that boosted my ego but deadened my spirit.

It wasn't uncommon for me to gaslight myself into believing that I alone was to blame for my suffering. I was constantly measuring myself to the impossible standards that were projected upon me by myself and my culture while falling woefully short, it seemed, at every turn.

At this rate, I would always be too much, and I would never be enough.

But alas, I was caught in the all too common collective cycle most women find themselves in at some point in their lives—the double bind of "good-girl" programming that keeps the majority of women in patriarchal society malnourished in body, mind, and spirit.

Without knowing this, I kept striving to prove myself. I learned to dutifully avoid conflict and to continually reach for the wrong thing to fill the void inside of me—the insatiable hunger to feel enough in a world that was never designed to approve or accept me.

So dissociated was I that I continually found myself in toxic relationships and friendships that would often end in disastrous ways, thereby providing additional evidence of my ineptitude and proclivity for poor choices.

Fractured in my ability to concentrate, chronically anxious, and eventually succumbing to illness, I would learn that 80% of American women suffer from chronic auto-immune conditions.

This diagnosis would undermine my health for years to come and would eventually be the proverbial straw that broke the camel's back.

Divorced, addicted, broke, trapped, overwhelmed, disconnected, and bound by chains I could not see, I felt desperate to be free.

Through religion, school, television, media, gender roles, and unexamined narratives and doctrines, I would learn from birth that females in cultures around the world are urged, molded, and manipulated at every turn to become handmaidens of patriarchal culture.

While this paradigm also victimizes men, women are systematically relegated to second-class citizenship. This leaves us in tragic states of imbalance, keeping the status quo in place and allowing the proliferation of power, profit, extraction, greed, and genocide to go unchecked and unchallenged. The longer we remain trapped in good-girl programming, the closer we get to losing it all.

Most women are horrified and stunned to learn that this particular brand of oppression, once revealed, is ancient, generational, pervasive, and relentless - a practice that has been in place for over 2,500 years and until now, has been hiding in plain sight. Like The Wizard of Oz, the man behind the curtain represents the illusions of patriarchy that are being revealed at a rapid pace as the poly-crisis continues to converge in what feels like a collective underworld experience.

The unstable and unsustainable systems that have propped up the patriarchal paradigm are finally crumbling, and the "good" girls are awakening to remember that our virtue was never the issue but a distraction to keep us preoccupied from knowing our true power.

We are UNBECOMING.

As centuries of generational oppression come crashing down, we must remember that it's not in our interest to uphold, manage, fix, or stop the destruction from happening. We must bear witness to its demise and hold each other through the change as we collectively endeavor to create a more beautiful world our hearts know is possible.

This is an opportunity to reject the old and create anew, but to do so, we must make space to unravel—to return home to our authentic and imperfect selves, which requires profound vulnerability.

Unbecoming is an invitation to strip off the illusions and step boldly into being who you are vs. what you think you should be.

This includes becoming full of ourselves - welcoming back the parts we have exiled and rediscovering what makes us come alive by giving ourselves a chance to live and love ourselves as we never have before.

It's a time of unbecoming from cultural codes of false virtue - for these have not kept us safe, happy, or whole, and we must process the toll of trauma that has kept us addicted to conflict with ourselves and others.

What does Unbecoming look like?

It looks different for everyone but for me it's about the inner child, those parts of me that never had a chance to express themselves, and resurrecting the inner artist, and the one who knows how to make magic and believes in miracles. The one who loves adventure and nature, and knows how to dance and play. The one who has the audacity to wear overalls again and whistle while painting in the sun.

It's about flirting with life and allowing myself pleasure and giving myself permission to say and do the things I've longed to experience.

It's about opting out of grind culture, taking time to smell the roses, and learning something new, simply because it brings me joy.

Collectively I think it's about Unbecoming from rigidity and fear by offering ourselves forgiveness and grace for the mistakes we've made along the way and daring to dream of a world we can't yet see.

It looks like Unbecoming from a savior complex because the freedom and spaciousness we seek will never come from an exterior source. We must seek and find within ourselves our selfhood, thereby

202

granting us permission to celebrate and approve of ourselves as we are- an important and vital part of this human story.

The heroine of this story is not content with the world as it is. In fact, her discontent and intolerance, her restlessness and determination—these seemingly unseemly qualities—ultimately become the source of her strength and redemption, sending her on the ultimate quest to uncover her truth.

This is a revolutionary and necessary time that requires us to become what patriarchal power has feared all along: the voices of activism and awareness. We become women who reach higher and higher octaves as more of us disrupt the status quo by speaking truth to power.

This is an epic time of unbecoming— a time to unriddle ourselves from who the world told us to be, to discover and reveal the truth of who we are- powerful and vital co-equal stewards of the Earth. We will no longer buy into the white supremacist colonial program of ecocide and genocide being enacted unchecked and unchallenged.

Do I see this as a time of great challenge? Yes. In our reclamation of the feminine, things will get messy and maybe even brutal. There will be destruction and collapse, for this is inevitable. There will be rage, sorrow, grief, and tears. And it is an opportunity to heal, discover, and redefine what it means to be human.

Is Unbecoming easy? Hell no.

But it's worth every moment and filled with more treasure along the way than you ever imagined.

I'm here with you, and I'm inviting you to become the most UNBECOMING YOU the Patriarchy has ever seen.

Join me.

We ride at dawn.

About Monica Rodgers

Monica Rodgers is a transformational and leadership coach, author, podcaster, inner medicine, and rites of passage practitioner. Monica founded The Revelation Project and The Revelation Project Podcast- an individual and holistic movement to disrupt the trance of unworthiness and lift the veils of personal illusion and cultural deception that keep us from remembering the truth of who we are.

"There is a fountain of youth: It is your mind, your talents, the creativity you bring to your life and the lives of people you love. When you learn to tap this source, you will truly have defeated age."

— Sophia Loren

www.ingramcontent.com/pod-product-compliance
Lightning Source LLC
Chambersburg PA
CBHW060512130626
46553CB00002B/467